MW01232712

Kink Magic
Sex Magic Beyond Vanilla

Advance Praise for
Kink Magic: Sex Magic Beyond Vanilla

In Kink Magic, Taylor Ellwood and Lupa bring an experienced and sensible approach to the oft-sensationalized subjects of kinky sexuality and magic, exploring each in its own right, and finding creative and effective ways to blend them. Both kink and magic can be scary and unpredictable affairs, but the authors' calm and protective influence helps the reader navigate, challenge, and harness the shadows of the psyche to do no less than transform reality. I highly recommend this book to anyone kinky or magical; if you're both, it's required reading.

--Jennifer Hunter, author of *Rites of Pleasure: Sexuality in Wicca and Neo-Paganism* and *Wicca For Lovers*

Kink Magic discusses the how you can use dominance, submission, humiliation, and various other "transgressive" states as sources of energy for magical work. Writing with rare clarity and admirable honesty, they explore the practical application of a variety of magical techniques to bondage, discipline, sado-masochism, and a wide range of other mindsets and tropisms, providing extensive examples of personal experiences from their own journal entries... Kink Magic may be kinky, but it goes a long way towards straightening out common misconceptions regarding sexual magic.

--Bill Whitcomb, author of *The Magician's Companion* and *The Magician's Reflection*

The intersection of kinky sex and practical magick; pleasure, pain, and spirituality. A place of abundant energy, emotion, and power. Lupa and Taylor explore and explain this intersection in a positive way for members of both the kinky and magickal communities, bridging a gap that for many should not exist.

--Mistress Milliscent, http://www.milliscent.com

Kink Magic is a gorgeously-written and thoughtfully complete manual for the (relatively common but not commonly discussed) convergence of magical spirituality and the kink lifestyle. Insofar as kink, a wide array of pertinent material is clearly laid out, including BDSM, bondage, fetishism, sadomasochism, and gender-play. For anyone who is curious about either the kink or magical-spiritual lifestyle, this book is key.

--Raven Digitalis, author of *Goth Craft: The Dark Side of Magickal Culture* and *Shadow Magick Compendium*

Written in a down to earth, easy to understand, warm and casual style, *Kink Magick* is a balancing act between dominance and submission and the erotic dance of the sacred spirit. Both share experiences and insights, ritual and sex, pain and pleasure, love, growth and their personal truths, powerful, raw and profound. It's the book I wish I'd written!

--Sylvana Silverwitch, aka Mistress Damiana DeViante; HPS, Sylvan Grove; Publisher, *Widdershins*

Lupa and Taylor have produced a multilayered, thought-provoking manual of multicultural kink. Magicians searching for new ideas, and kinksters hungry for a deeper level to their scening will find much food for thought. You will get offended, you will get defensive, and you will come out the other side much better for it.

--Nicholas Graham, author of *The Four Powers: Magical Practice for Beginners of All Ages*

Kink Magic
Sex Magic Beyond Vanilla

Taylor Ellwood and Lupa

Megalithica books

Stafford, England

Kink Magic: Sex Magic Beyond Vanilla
Taylor Ellwood and Lupa
© 2007 First edition

http://www.thegreenwolf.com
http://www.kinkmagic.com

Cover Art: Naryu
Cover Design: Andy Bigwood
Internal Illustration: Daven
Editor: Sheta Kaey
Copy Editor: Nicholas Graham
Layout: Lupa

Set in Book Antiqua and Poor Richard

Megalithica Books Edition 2007

A Megalithica Books Publication
http://www.immanion-press.com
info@immanion-press.com

8 Rowley Grove
Stafford ST17 9BJ
UK

ISBN 978-1-905713-11-0

Dedication

To my amazing and lovely mate, Taylor, for being such an integral part of my life, and teaching me that I'm so much more than I thought I was. And to every partner I've ever had the pleasure of scening with, thank you for giving me those experiences and helping me feel more comfortable in my skin. Finally, I want to thank everyone who has been brave enough to fly their freak flags high, letting the world know that you can be entirely unconventional and still be a good person. --Lupa

To my lovely Lupa, who provides me the safest space of all, whether we're scening or not. You continue to show me that I can be more than I ever thought I could be. To every other partner, thank you for the privilege you gave me in allowing me to scene with you. Finally to all other people who choose to be true to themselves instead of to what other people think. It takes more courage to be yourself than to conform. --Taylor

Acknowledgements

Many thanks to Sheta for her awesome editing job, and to Nick for the clean copy edit. Mad appreciation also goes out to Dan and Dawn, and Daven for the guest essays, and Dossie Easton for the foreword. And many thanks to the good folks who previewed the work for blurbs and feedback. We would also like to thank the good folks on Livejournal who have been so supportive to us throughout this project. And we appreciate everyone who has given us venues to present workshops at, with a special thanks to Robert and Raven at the Edge of the Circle, the best occult book shop in Seattle, WA.

The CYA Page

Okay, folks, it's disclaimer time. This book contains material which may be hazardous to your health, the health of others, and if found may result in awkward confrontations by family, friends, coworkers, or police searching your home. Additionally, duplicating some of the exercises and other material may result in physical and/or psychological harm. Neither the authors nor the publisher are responsible in any way, shape, or form for any decisions, thoughts, or actions that you may take as a result of reading this book and/or using material found within it.

Some of the material here is *not* meant for novices in either BDSM or magic; if this is your first exposure to either of these practices, we recommend (in addition to the introductory chapters on both kink and magic) that you check out our bibliography for a really nice selection of both complementary and contrasting viewpoints. Our book is not exhaustive and should not be taken as a 101 course; we include our interpretations of 101 materials for contextual purposes only. We also strongly suggest that if you aren't involved in either of these communities that you make connections in at least one; there's sufficient crossover that you'll probably find people who are a part of both. Books are no substitute for interactions with real people (and no, we don't just mean getting laid!).

Depending on where you're reading this, this book may also be considered offensive and/or inappropriate, particularly for those under the age of 18. That being said, we are wholehearted proponents of the First Amendment to the United States Constitution, particularly these fine words:

Congress shall make no law...abridging the freedom of speech, or of the press.

We thank you for reading our words, whether in this book or others, and supporting everyone's freedom of speech. For, as Lupa has said on a number of occasions:

Your freedom of speech is my freedom of speech; the silencing of my voice sets the precedent that will in turn silence yours.

Table of Contents

Foreword

You are holding in your hands the best book about magic I have ever read, and the most amazing journey between two people that I have ever been allowed into. Lupa and Taylor Ellwood share practice and understanding of magic with the reader with utter lucidity and clarity.

Do you believe in magic? I suppose that depends on what we think magic is. Forgot about Cinderella's fairy godmother, although we do admit that costumes are indeed a way of traveling in magic, when we make the costumes ourselves, as ways of trying on being different from how we have been before. Magic, you see, is a way of traveling in your mind--your entire mind, not just the easy parts.

And magic is a way of moving stuff around in your mind, a chance to rearrange your mental furniture: why is that old footstool right inside the door where I keep stubbing my toe on it? Maybe we could banish it to the attic until somebody finds a better use for it.

What is exciting about this is that there is now and always will be more of the mind, more of the self to explore and to welcome into consciousness. We are not going to run out of new frontiers within ourselves or in our energetic connections with each other and with the Divine Unity of the Universe. Kink magicians focus energy raised from ritual, power exchange, intense stimulations and, yes please, sex and sensuality, to delve into questions and conflicts, to find new answers within themselves that enlarge their knowledge and capacity, and enable them to grasp their personal power and free them to be ever more themselves.

Why sex magic? Why not? I am more surprised to realize that it is possible to have sex that isn't magic, albeit probably not very much fun. When we journey into our sexual states of consciousness, we leave ordinary reality behind and travel in extraordinary joy and connection, with the capacity to flow into ecstatic and transcendent states of mind. Working magic then becomes the application of intention to that already magic journey. We can enjoy sex and sensuality purely for the magic wonder of it, or we can take it a step further and seek, in that exalted state of mind, answers to our problems and pathways to further expansion and deeper self-awareness.

This book approaches magic as something we can all learn, with due respect for the need to learn something. When we are willing to study ritual paths and understand how to make it safe to dance down them, we can all be magicians.

When we bring together ritual and sexuality, we are already wandering into kink. Because kink is not some weird stuff that is only enjoyed by people who are broken or bent or *different*; kink, being perfectly natural, is where expanded sexual exploration tends to lead. In many ways, kink already is ritual, as the roles we play of victims and villains, angels, demons and so on, constitute the bringing into reality of archetypal energies sometimes conceived of as gods and goddesses, other times understood as psychodrama. Doesn't matter a lot what you call it as long as we are prepared for the truth that in the psychodrama of kink ritual mythic journeys are undertaken. Driven by the vehicles of intense physical stimulations; the giving and receiving of various forms of personal power; and the whole script animated, injected and enthused with the healing juice of Eros. Goody!

Taylor and Lupa teach us that "a BDSM lifestyle exists to create an exchange of power without effect on the outside world" where no one is stealing power from anyone else, or trying to bolster their own power at someone else's expense, but rather power is handed back and forth for ritual purpose or delight, with the ultimate goal that both or all parties are further empowered.

In the chapters on Metamorphic Magic, we are educated about the uses of BDSM ritual to heal and transform, wherein roleplay becomes invocation, and costume an invitation for some mysterious part of ourselves to come out and play. Many of these are dark journeys, into pain and shame, difficult histories, or just plain stuck places in ourselves. Part of the magic of kink is that when we delve into our own shame and infuse it with Eros, perhaps intensifying it with orgasm, we can transform pain into compassion and humiliation into pride.

So Lupa and Taylor show us what happens when we add intention to exploration, ask a question of a quest or explore a troubled feeling as if it were a gateway. We can bind ourselves to our journey with ropes and chains while our beloveds drive us out of our everyday minds with whips and canes and we open our hearts to the Cosmos as we open our skin to sharp sharp steel ... and return from all this excitement to drop back into loving arms and snuggle or weep while we learn how to fit into this new self we have discovered.

You have in your hands a wonderful guidebook for these kinds of journeys. Lupa and Taylor offer up the wisdom of many years of brave explorations of their psyches, and they generously share their personal experiences--the easy and the not-necessarily-quite-so easy--from all the paths they have walked or danced or crawled down together in quest of ownership of more of themselves.

This book is full of adventures into the inner wilderness, and down to earth info on how to travel safely in our precious inner jungles. One trait that draws me into this work is that the authors don't ask us to believe anything in particular--there is no dogma here, only possibilities to check out. They relate their own journeys with wondrous generosity, to show us how they use kink energy to delve into themselves, access their wisdom and travel together fearlessly in love. I am in awe of what they have built in their relationship. As I read about their intense and intimate connections I must admit to some envy of their loving and magical partnership. I hope it will inspire me to build more of such partnerships into my own life.

Thank you, Taylor, thank you, Lupa, for bravely bringing such wisdom into our lives.

Dossie Easton
Co-author with Janet Hardy of *Radical Ecstasy*
9/10/2007

Introduction

There are a lot of kinky magicians, and a lot of magical kink fans. In fact, for many people the two go as well together as...well...*better* than peanut butter and jelly. The translation from one to the other is relatively simple when things like altered states of consciousness and ritualized psychodrama are taken into account. We've met, both as a couple and as individuals, in person and online, hundreds of people who are into both practices, and as sales of recent books on this wonderful mixture have shown, there's plenty more where they came from! With growing acceptance of kink and magic, more people feel comfortable exploring their taboo interests and will likely experience the same realization that we, other authors, and numerous other people have known for a while — that kink and magic work quite nicely in tandem.

Please keep in mind that this is our personal approach to non-vanilla sex magic. There are as many ways to be kinky as there are kinky people, and as many ways to practice magic as there are magicians. The strength of any topic, when it comes to written literature, lies in the variety of voices offered. Our goal is to provide a unique perspective on the topic that is primarily practical rather than spiritual in content. The majority of excellent books we've found tend to treat kink magic as more of a spiritual path to honor the gods, or to travel to other planes of reality. While we touch on these ideas from our own perspectives, our primary purpose is to provide the reader with practical exercises and rituals meant to deliberately manifest reality both macrocosmically and microcosmically — in other words, practical magic.

We approach this topic more as magicians than kinky folk, though both aspects of our lives are important to this work. While both of us have been decidedly *not* vanilla as long as we've been sexual people, we don't have the involvement with the BDSM and fetish Scene that we do with the pagan and occult communities; our interaction with other kinky people comes from friends and acquaintances who just happen to be kinky already. That's not to say that we ignore other kinky folk, or that we'll continue in this pattern forever. However, we're writing as magicians who are integrating kink into magic, rather than kinky people who are integrating magic into our play.

For us, magic is about flexibility and change as well as manifesting desire into reality, and this permeates our entire worldview. It should come as no surprise that we view our kink similarly. You'll notice in a few pages, for instance, that the first example we give in this book talks about a mild D/S relationship with Lupa as the dominant and Taylor as the submissive. That particular anecdote stems from early in our relationship and practice together; it was the dynamic that best fit our situation at the time, both as a couple and as individuals. Since then we've both evolved into full-time switches, taking whatever roles are needed and desired at a particular time. We both have collars given to us by the other, and there are times when we both wear them as a sign of commitment and service to each other. That doesn't mean that our D/S stage wasn't genuine, or that "switch" is the permanent or "natural" alignment for both of us. Humans are mutable, and we embrace what works best for us at any given point in our lives.

If you happen to be familiar with our other works, it may seem a little strange for us to have basic chapters on kink and magic since we have a tendency to avoid 101 material. Because we're covering two different areas of theory and practice here we can't assume that every reader will already have a working knowledge of both. For those who have little to no experience in one or both of these topics, we wanted to give some background material for clarification of our work as a whole. Additionally, we've added this material for author-specific context. The ways that we understand and use both kink and magic are unique to us, just as your applications of these are specifically yours, so we added these chapters to give you some context for later material. If you're a novice to kink or magic, we recommend reading other books on these subjects as well as networking with more knowledgeable people before using the material in this book. While we allude to basic magical techniques and features of BDSM, our primary how-tos involve the more advanced work of kink magic itself.

We do make references to other books we've written, as other authors often do. Sadly, this is often cynically interpreted as the authors attempting to self-promote. While nobody would argue over selling more books, in our case at least we do this to offer people a heads-up that we've written more extensively on certain topics elsewhere. Rather than repeat ourselves from book to book, we instead point out where people who are interested in these concepts may find out more information without stuffing the pages of this book with rehashed material.

We're not going to spoon-feed you a bunch of prefabricated rituals. Our offerings here consist of the elements of kink magic, discussion of techniques, and ideas to help you to create scenes and rituals of your own. We illustrate these things with anecdotes from our own experimentation as well as some more in-depth explanations of specific rites we've done, but we don't expect you to duplicate every single one to the tiniest little detail. If you're inspired by our examples, great! Take the ideas and run with them. But were we to give you a book full of nothing but step-by-step rituals that we wrote, it would go against the individuality of kink magic.

Okay. Now that you know where we're coming from, let us show you where we're going...

Chapter One: What is Kink Magic?
December 26, 2005 – From the Journal of Lupa

When I first started learning about magic, my primary exposure was through neopaganism. This immersion involved a fairly high rate of white light ethics. My introduction to the concept of binding magic was as a way to get rid of people or energies that were problematic. The idea was to restrict the person/energy so that the influence on you was either lessened or altered. In any case, it was one of the few times in which having control over someone other than yourself was acceptable.

Fast forward a few years, to this past week. At this point, my mate Taylor and I have a mild, laid-back BDSM lifestyle; I am the dominant and he is my submissive. It's not so much a matter of me beating the hell out of him if he doesn't wash the dishes every day as it is that he knows that doing the dishes will please me, and that it's his place to do so. I allow him to express his complete devotion to me in any manner he sees fit, even in mundane ways. While we take turns topping each other, I am the definite dominant — I call the shots in the relationship, by mutual agreement (and sometimes sheer spoiled bitchiness). We can be unconventional, but it works for us.

We recently got to the point where I decided to gift him with a collar. I didn't want to use it as a way of signifying ownership, so much as I wanted to give him something that would symbolize my care and protection of him in return for his devotion. So it was off to one of the local fetish shops where lovely handmade toys and things could be purchased for reasonable rates. We picked out a leather collar with a D-ring, something we both agreed was definitely "him".

Taylor had expressed to me previously that he'd wanted me to bind him magically--I'm a definite switch, but had always seemed to end up with people who for various reasons didn't want anything to do with bottoming or subbing. Taylor began to slowly introduce me to the idea of my being not only a top but a dominant, and once I got over my initial "You mean I actually get to *do* that?" shock I took to it nicely.

So by the time he started asking me about magical binding as part of our D/S, I was quite happy to consider it as a way to please him. After all, while the submissive may seem to be getting the short end of the stick, it really **is** a two-way street. Unless you're in a really *extreme* lifestyle (which we're not), both/all parties in a D/S relationship need to be satisfied and happy in order for it to be healthy (though there are people who enjoy being frustrated and nearly abused in some very drastic ways). I decided that the collar would be the perfect vehicle for the binding magic, as it symbolized not only his commitment to care for me and serve me, but also my commitment to protect and care for him. In addition, I made the caveat that he did not have to consult me if he wanted to remove the collar, and therefore the binding; I wanted a creature of free will, not broken will.

When we got home from the fetish shop, I pulled out the Alphabet of Desire I designed a while back. It's a series of lines and whorls that correlate to the 26 letters of the English alphabet that I use for magical purposes. I composed a sentence that I felt more than sufficiently spoke my desire, and sigilized each word using my AoD. I then painted it in silver acrylic on the front of the collar, with one half of the words on one side of the D-ring and the rest on the other side.

On the night we did the final ritual, I was at the greatest flow of my menstrual period. I took him into our ritual area and made him sit on the cloth reserved for sex magic while I prepared the ritual area.

Our D/S dynamic takes a bit of inspiration from wolfpack structures as perceived through human understanding. We're hardly the first people to do this, but I'm very strongly wolf-identified; Wolf is my primary totem, and I've adopted a number of lupine aspects and symbols (though, thankfully, no attraction to anything but *Homo sapiens*!). I first adopted him as "pack." I invoked Wolf into me and then passed that energy to him, giving him a permanent piece of my lupine self and thereby a connection to the totem Wolf. Before I could be Alpha to his Beta, I first wanted to acknowledge him as being Pack. In doing so, I stated that although he was my submissive, he was still equally important in the end-- hence my commitment to care for him and protect him even as he does the same for me in different ways. After all, an actual wolf pack is nowhere near as militaristic or hierarchical as humans sometimes project, and involves much more fluidity than is often assumed. Additionally, in the words of Kipling, "The strength of the Pack is the Wolf, and the strength of the Wolf is the Pack". Taylor might have been submissive to me, but he wasn't a lesser being (hence our use of a capital S in D/S, as opposed to the usual lower case s).

Still, I wanted to show him his place in my pack in a dramatic manner that would imprint on his psyche. I threw him to the floor and pinned him with my body, then fucked him, and allowed the energy that the blood gave to open up and flow through me. The blood served as a strong psychological and magical representation of my power over him, both in its inherent magical qualities and in the strong taboos that have existed in many cultures banning a person from sleeping with a menstruating partner (in heterosexual situations). While it's not necessarily something that would work with every situation, it was quite the effective enhancement to this particular ritual.

I used the energy raised during sex to further bind him to me. I visualized my own energy streaming out of my body, latching onto his energy and becoming a number of ropes that wrapped around his limbs and his body, secure but not so tight as to be cumbersome. They became thicker and stronger as we each neared climax, the event of which made the bindings permanent as I poured everything we both had into them.

Once we both caught our breath and returned to our skins, I anointed the collar with a tiny amount of our mixed sexual fluids, blood and all, in between the two layers of leather, and placed it around his neck. It now serves as a physical reminder of the bindings I placed upon him. Because of the nature of its making, it can't be used against me, but as with any submissive's or slave's collar, it's a tool of control; the magic simply enhances that control many times. And, as stated previously, if he becomes uncomfortable with the D/S aspect of our relationship, there's nothing preventing him from removing the collar and the magic until we can work things out.

Taylor Speaks:

I find strong women to be an incredible turn-on, particularly those willing to show a man his proper subservient place. The idea of having a magical binding placed on me by a dominant female magician also really appeals to me, probably because my first encounter with a dominant woman involved a magician who bound me to keep me aware of her, even long after the relationship was over.

Don't get me wrong; I'm well aware of what a binding is. It's a constraining of someone, a binding to the will of another. In most situations, I wouldn't be for it at all, but in a close relationship with a committed partner, I felt comfortable giving that level of control. I knew that it would be a test of what I was willing to accept and submit to, and that appealed to me. Finally, I trusted Lupa. We have excellent communication between us, and I never felt like she would take advantage of such a binding.

The night of the binding was preceded by several days of really thinking about the commitment I was going to undertake. The night we bought the collar, I wore it so I could really feel it and think about what it meant. But the next day I had to leave to pack my belongings, as I was scheduled to move into her place, and I had to leave the collar behind and spend a day without it. I was able to contemplate what it felt like not to have a collar and what that meant to me. The day without the collar was hard, because I realized I really did want to accept and wear it. I also realized that it wasn't my choice. If I was to wear one, it would be at her pleasure, in her time, not my own.

When I drove back to her place, I anticipated a life-changing experience. I knew I wanted the collar. I knew I wanted to be with her, and putting on that collar was a commitment to her. I got home (for now her place really was my home as well) and waited. When she got home from work and saw me there, we agreed it was time to do the ritual.

After a shower, she had me sit on a red mat. I waited there, head bowed, as she made the room ready for the ritual. When she put the wolf spirit into me and then seized me and took me, I felt helpless. I could feel the binding energy wrap around my limbs and neck. When she anointed the collar with our fluids and put it around my neck, the binding was sealed. I knew I belonged to her in a way I had never belonged to anyone. Not only were my body and mind bound to her will, but my spirit was as well. The magic I could do was bound to her wishes. This was done freely, of my choice, but it was also a submission of that choice to her.

Later in our relationship, the dynamic changed. We got out of the D/S context and both became switches. But I still have the collar, and when I feel submissive I wear it as a reminder of the service that has been granted to me by her. When I take the collar off, the binding is not active, for it's tied into the collar itself. Yet every time I put on that collar, I feel that binding energy on me and I know I am bound to her so long as I wear the collar. It's a binding of submission, but also of perfect love and perfect trust (or as close to perfect as you can reasonably get), which are some of the most potent magical forces any person can work with.

Historical Perspectives

The ritual we've just described is just one example of the ways in which BDSM and other kinks can be woven into effective magical practice—and vice versa. This isn't a new concept. Kink has been a part of human sexuality and psychology for millennia. One early example can be found on a Greek cup dating over 500 years before the birth of Christ. Etched in the familiar black-on-earth colors of this period are figures engaged in orgiastic scenes—proof that pornography isn't a new phenomenon! Along with several different sexual acts and positions, some of the participants are shown wielding implements of possible pain infliction, including a trident and an instrument that looks either like a horn or possibly a flail. Several of the couplings/triads have a suggestion of power play about them in the way the bodies are positioned and the manner in which the person receiving the penetration is held and manipulated by the penetrators (Néret 2005). A circa 1514 work that Marc-Antoine Raimondi did, based on Raphael, shows two satyrs kidnapping a nude woman. The captive is draped over the back and shoulders of one, while it appears that the other is preparing to level a blow to her backside (Néret 2005).

While these scenes may or may not have been intended to be suggestive in such a kinky manner, later works of erotic art were most decidedly non-vanilla. An illustration for John Cleland's *Fanny Hill or Memoirs of a Woman of Pleasure* dating from the second half of the 18th century features a whipping scene (Néret 2005). Not long after this made its debut, Count Donatien Alphonse Francois de Sade began living out his fantasies—as well as writing them down. Among his works were *Justine* and *Juliette*, and all were filled with graphic descriptions of sadomasochism. These were deemed perverted enough at the time that they ultimately helped to land him in prison, from whence he published his famous novels on sadistic practices. In the following century, Leopold von Sacher-Masoch wrote *Venus in Furs*, an exploration of pain-filled submission that led to his name evolving into the term *masochism* (Wallechinsky & Wallace 1975).

Kinky erotica is well-known, but pain and power play in historical magic and religion is a less-published topic. Probably the most famous examples are the religious flagellants, particularly those associated with Catholic monasticism, which dated back as far as the 13th century (Toke 1909). One particularly notable example was St. Mary Magdalene de Pazzi, who was canonized in 1671. Not only did she self-flagellate religiously, but she would also strip herself naked and roll on thorns and other sharp objects. She even tried getting her fellow nuns into the act, attempting to convince them to bind her and then participate in a little holy wax play with her. At one point when she was helping newcomers to the convent get settled into the routine, she managed to get one of them to flog her (Wallechinsky & Wallace 1978). There were other, more organized examples as well. These included, among others, the Khlysti, a Russian cult that Rasputin was allegedly part of, who used a Christian framework (Dawn & Flowers 2001).

Christianity hardly has the monopoly on spiritual pain. Zoroastrianism, one of the precursors to Christianity, featured a flogging for purification prior to certain sacrifices. The Lakota Sun Dance involved piercing the muscles of the chest and then using the piercings to hang the participants to induce trance states. The Mediterranean region was also home to a number of religious traditions that donated religious whipping to Greek and Roman celebrations. An example was the Spartan "feast of flagellations" in which youths were whipped in public as a form of sacrifice. A later incarnation of this practice was the fertility-magic-laden flail of Lupercalia, used on young women to help encourage procreation (in more ways than one, perhaps!) (Dawn & Flowers 2001).

Kink Magic Today

Kink magic, as we define it, uses principles and practices of BDSM and sexual fetish in magical practice. The primary purpose of kink magic is to manifest desire into reality and to create change on a conscious, though not always physical, level. Kink provides the means to focus both the top and bottom on the desired goal, while magic provides the method for directing the focused energies into the manifestation of the desire.

We divide magic into practical and metamorphic. Practical magic includes tangible results, such as charging a sigil for a successful business venture, or performing a ritual to attract suitable partners (but not specific people, which is not only considered by many to be unethical, but also severely limits your potential dating/etc. pool). Metamorphic magic, on the other hand, can be anything from a pathworking utilizing the Kabbalistic Tree of Life to invoking aspects of yourself in order to shatter your ego-driven tunnel vision. Practical magic creates mainly external change, while the domain of metamorphic magic is primarily internal.

Kink works in nicely in the altered states of consciousness it creates. An altered state of conscious (ASC) is one that differs in a significant way from your "normal," everyday state of consciousness (ESC). (Remember those two acronyms — we'll be using them a lot.) It provides a wonderful psychodrama to rival any traditional ceremony, and trains people to access parts of themselves that they normally leave in the background. Additionally, the application of pain releases chemicals into the body which help to bring the recipient to new levels of awareness. No wonder, then, that so many people find kink magic to be a highly effective practice![1]

In the Event You're Feeling Uncomfortable...

You're almost through the first chapter. How are you feeling?

If you're enjoying this and looking forward to the rest of the book, you probably already know most (if not all) of what's in this final section. On the other hand, we accept that some people might be a little (or a lot) uncomfortable with kink, magic, or both. It's the latter group that we'd like to address for a moment.

There are a lot of misconceptions about both kink and magic outside of these two subcultures. Both tend to be highly sensationalized by the media and are easy targets for political and religious leaders looking to whip up...errr...inflame the passions of...ah...get people excited about...um. Well, needless to say, they're trying to evoke the emotions of their respective constituents and congregations, and both minority religions and "weird" sex practices are targets.

Unfortunately, few of these people ever really talk to members of either subculture. America in particular is based on a dualistic model of thinking which requires a definite good/evil, black/white split in order to feel somewhat secure. Add in any note of ambiguity and people panic. Sympathy for the perceived devil is seen as a weakness of faith and morals, which means that those who are demonized rarely get a chance to speak for themselves. This

---

[1] Even modern science is finding that pain can be therapeutic; a 2005 study in Russia found that patients with everything from substance addiction to depression showed improvement in their outlooks after being whipped on the butt, particularly when administered by a member of the opposite sex. (Anonymous, 2005)

makes establishing dialogues difficult, and getting accurate information that isn't full of exaggerations and outright lies is sometimes challenging.

Fortunately, over the past couple of decades there have been a number of brave souls who have worked to improve P.R. for the kink and pagan communities. Both individuals and organizations have stepped forward to demonstrate that we aren't all sexual predators and devil-worshippers sacrificing your cat in the nearest grave yard. Others have been unwillingly thrust into the spotlight, losing jobs or custody battles over personal choices that people made assumptions about.

Think of the most lurid stereotypes you can about kinky people and pagans. "Sadomasochists are all sick rapists and victims." "Pagans spit on Christianity." Sound familiar? Maybe you've got even worse ones in mind. Chances are, though, that they're not true for the vast majority of people in a given subculture. There may be a few people way out on the fringes who resemble these remarks, but they find themselves ostracized from their respective communities as well as the mainstream. Smear campaigns are as old as human society itself, and pulling out the most negative examples of a group to display as the norm is a common practice.

That doesn't make it true, though. Abuse does happen in the kink community, and there are some very anti-Christian pagans out there. That doesn't mean that either the former or the latter are the rule rather than the exception. We have each been involved with pagans and kinky people for years, and the vast majority of people in both groups that we've encountered have been harmless, respectful people with "normal" lives. The average pagan or kinky person has a day job, a family, a healthy social life, and a clean criminal record, just like anyone else. We just happen to have different beliefs and/or practices.

We hope that by reading this book you can get a little better idea of what we're talking about and why it appeals to us. As with any paradigm, though, it's important to have a solid grounding in specific material – after all, you couldn't perform ceremonial magic with no knowledge of the tools, rites and techniques specific to it. Kink is a wide category, just as magic is, with a lot of territory to cover. In the next two chapters, we're going to go over the basics of both kink and magic as we understand them. Again, we recommend reading beyond this book if you haven't already; check out the bibliography for further reading material.

And if you're still looking rather askance at this book, may we suggest just putting it down? You can let the material you have read digest a bit, and come back to it when you're feeling better. Or you can walk away entirely and never look back--whatever works best for you. We just ask that you give it a fair, relatively objective chance rather than automatically judging it according to whatever biases you've brought in.

Chapter Two: The Principles of Kink

Kink involves a whole wide world of sexual fetishism and play. A fetish, in the original sexual sense, is an object or action without which a person absolutely cannot become aroused; for example, BDSM in general may be a fetish for a person who simply isn't turned on physically without it[2]. These days the meaning has been relaxed a bit, becoming synonymous with anything that is outside the pale of commonly acceptable sex practices, though it may simply add spice to sex rather than being necessary for it to occur.

Those "acceptable" practices, what are often referred to by kinky folk as "vanilla," involve sex that generally doesn't include deliberate pain, power play, or fetishes not generally accepted by mainstream society. Vanilla is actually a very narrow category, depending on how fluid you allow the boundaries to be. Is a couple who may indulge in a bit of playful spanking before sex kinky or vanilla? How about those who hold their partners' wrists above their heads during sex, but not in any sort of deliberate context? Is doggy style kinky or vanilla? Regardless of where the lines are drawn, vanilla leaves a lot of territory for kink to play in.

While BDSM is the most common association with kink, they may be mutually exclusive; in a Venn diagram, BDSM would be a circle within a larger circle labeled "kink", which itself would mostly (but not entirely) overlap the "fetish" circle. A man who likes to wear women's underwear may do so for a purely sensual experience, rather than the perceived humiliation of forced feminization. Additionally, some fetishes may be considered vanilla because they're more or less acceptable among the general populace. Obsession with and idealization of breasts, asses, and legs on women, and well-toned muscles on men, are thoroughly woven into the majority of society's (mostly hetero) sexuality. Kink assumes some level of unacceptability by the cultural status quo, something that these nearly universal fetishes clearly avoid (other than via moralistic religious fundamentalists who think all sex is wrong!).

---

[2] The use of the word "fetish" in a kinky sense should not be confused with the use of the term in the magical sense, at least insofar as indigenous cultures go. Otherwise, as Lupa once quipped, "Then there's the Zuni fetish, which involves being turned on by a person on hands and knees with a zigzagged arrow painted down hir side and a stone arrow tied to hir back."

Kink doesn't necessarily involve the sexual act itself, either. There are plenty of people, for example, who will play with others to a certain point, but may draw the line at oral, anal, and/or vaginal sex. Others may scene all the way to sex one time, and only to a certain point the next. Sometimes it depends on the people involved and what their relationship to each other is; other times it hinges on setting. Sex is a no-no at a public dungeon. However, a play party may or may not be sex-friendly depending upon who's hosting it. Obviously, if you're in the privacy of your own home and you don't live with anyone who'd be agitated by your actions, anything goes.

In the next few pages, we're going to explore some of the more common categories of kink. We're not going to go too in-depth, as there are already a number of really good books devoted solely to kink techniques, which we've listed in the bibliography and other recommended reading. Nor are we going to integrate every single fetish we discuss into kink magic — some of these are, quite simply, Not Our Kink. For example, while we realize that some people really, *really* get into playing with urine and feces on a sexual level, and you can certainly integrate it into your kink magic if that's your kink, that particular area of interest is NOK, so we won't actually have any examples of magical urophilia and coprophilia in this book. We're just going to introduce the concepts to give you an idea of how broad a topic kink really is!

BDSM

The acronym stands for bondage, discipline, sadism, and masochism; the D and S also allude to dominance and submission. It's sort of an umbrella for several areas of kink — sadism and masochism, power play, and bondage and discipline. BDSM players may only choose to use some of these elements; it isn't necessary to use them all at once to be practicing "true" BDSM. In addition, people who indulge in these sorts of play may not even use the BDSM label.

The term "edgeplay" is used to describe activities that carry a (comparative) lot of health risks, such as knife play, fire play, or electrical play, or pushes people deep into their psyche, as with extreme humiliation. Edgeplay can be purely physical, as in whipping a person to the point of (or beyond) the safe word, or it can involve the breaking down of a person into utter and complete complacency. Edgeplay pushes the limits of one or both partners. What is edgeplay for one person may be nearly vanilla for another, and opinions about what constitutes edgeplay within the general BDSM community may vary over time as some practices become more acceptable.

"Scene" has a dual meaning within BDSM, referring either to a single bout of play between partners, or the BDSM/kink community as a whole. The latter Scene is often given an uppercase "s" and is composed of both public dungeons and gatherings, and more private parties, as well as informational meetings, munches and seminars. You don't have to be a part of the community to practice BDSM, however. In fact, some of the people we know who are into BDSM rarely, if ever, participate in formal events. The decreasing reliance on the community as the only safe space available seems to partly be due to the fact that compared to several decades ago, BDSM is now relatively more acceptable. We know quite a few people who have been comfortably kinky for as long as they've been sexual, and they've never seen it as anything less matter-of-fact than vanilla. Part of this is due to the groundwork that the community laid in making BDSM more acceptable. However, the sheer increase in available information is also a large factor. The quantity and quality of books has grown in recent years, and the internet, of course, has spawned countless numbers of informational websites of varying qualities, along with forums, chat rooms and other vectors of conversation. Still, there's something to be said about going to a play party or dungeon and watching other people do their thing, as well as trading notes at more informal, informational meetings. Books—even this one—can only do so much, and don't replace flesh-and-blood people.

Bondage

While bondage is the "B" in BDSM, there are bondage purists who dislike the D, S, and M. For them, being bound isn't about being "tortured" or dominated, but is for the sheer sense of restriction. Some people even find that being bound brings a feeling of security rather than fear. On the other hand, bondage of some sort is a mainstay of BDSM, hence its inclusion in the acronym.

The most common image of bondage involves leather cuffs, collars, and maybe even chains. Ropes are popular, too, though certain types work better (and are safer!) than others. *Screw the Roses, Send Me the Thorns* by Philip Miller and Molly Devon has some good basic information on rope bondage. Japanese rope bondage is particularly aesthetically pleasing, designed not only to bind a person but also show hir body off. Clamps for nipples, clits, and other body parts, as well as carefully applied clothespins, may also be considered forms of bondage, especially when attached to thin chains or strings and used to delicately immobilize a person. Leather cuffs[3] are almost clichéd in BDSM, and just being able to bind a person's wrists together will still restrict motion and make hir more pliable for other activities. People with healthy finances may be able to purchase more elaborate forms of bondage equipment, like spanking benches or St. Andrew's Crosses, or may build them themselves if they're so inclined.

Sometimes the best form of bondage doesn't involve anything but the people themselves. We're particularly fond of body bondage, in which one of us will pin the other, either with joint locks or sheer strength or getting a good (but careful!) grip on more, ah, delicate parts of the anatomy. In addition, psychological bondage is effective when control has already been firmly made clear. The person being bound is told to hold a particular position, upon threat of dire punishment (even if it's understood rather than stated). Finally, there is also energetic bondage, where energy work is used to restrain or even drain a person of the ability to resist.

Discipline

Discipline is all about psychology. Remember when you got in trouble as a kid? Depending on your parents' style of raising children, you may have been yelled at, spanked, or grounded. Regardless of how you were punished, though, it wasn't at all effective if it didn't work psychologically. Your parents might have belted the hell out of you for anything you did wrong, but if it didn't intimidate you, you may have grown even more headstrong—just the opposite of the desired effect. Or, if grounded, you might simply have sneaked out the window at night.

Discipline is similar in kink. Proper discipline involves psychologically molding a sub/slave/et al to obedience. While it

---

[3] Metal handcuffs, even furry ones, are generally not recommended. They can injure the wrists, which have a lot of nerves and blood vessels close to the surface, as they're not particularly flexible. Additionally, if you lose the key or if the lock jams they're not as easy to cut off as rope or leather. Finally, some areas may restrict civilian ownership of hand and ankle cuffs.

may consist of inflicting pain and binding hir physically, the crucial factor is all in the head. Discipline is designed to program the sub/etc. to behave in a certain manner while scening (or 24/7 if in a lifestyle situation).

Some people don't care for a lot of discipline. For example, both of us love willful bottoms who will put up a good fight rather than just rolling over and playing dead at the drop of a flogger. Other people, though, may prefer to be (or have) perfectly trained slaves ready to serve as toys, servants or footstools.

S/M and D/S

The sadist enjoys inflicting pain; quite often, it is a true fetish. The masochist is hir counterpart, enjoying the "tender attentions" that the sadist metes out. (Of course, there's the old joke, "What's the difference between a masochist and a sadist? The masochist says 'hurt me!' and the sadist says 'no!'".) A person may be one, the other, or both. The pain may be a light pinch, or it may push the masochist to hir limits—and there are all the delightful points in between.

In their purest forms, sadism and masochism are physical manifestations; there's no need for any psychological play along with it. However, the majority of their fans tend to also use power play/dominance and submission (D/S). This is a formalized, consensual exchange of power between two (or more) people. It may or may not include bondage and discipline; its manifestations are highly individualized. Some people keep it within a single scene; others make a lifestyle about it. D/S can be something as subtle as a forced kiss, or it may involve objectifying someone to the point where they are reduced to the level of a piece of furniture. The control may be exchanged without a fight, or there may be a mock struggle. Control can even change within a scene if both partners are flexible enough at switching.

24/7 Lifestyles and Total Power Exchange (TPE)

D/S relationships vary in intensity. While for many people, D/S is limited primarily to scenes; for others, it's a constant part of their lives. The manifestations of this vary; in many, though not all, cases, the people involved live together (or at least in the same area).

However, long distance situations aren't unheard of, though they may require a bit more creativity in their execution.

The parameters of the lifestyle vary as well. Some people restrict the overt displays for the bedroom and/or fetish events. Others actively exercise the power dynamic all the time at home, and in more subtle ways in public. In private or safe space, the submissive may serve the dominant, perform household chores or submit to the dominant's demands of varying types. Public displays of affection in this situation can range from the use of certain words designed to have specific effects, to a gentle tug on a collar/choker or clothing, and even particular expressions. This all depends on the individual relationship.

Some people are involved in total power exchange (TPE). While the "total" can never literally be achieved, TPE participants work to be as close to that as possible. This is where master/slave arrangements are typically found; every decision in the slave's life is turned over to the master/mistress; some go so far as to place all financial and legal responsibility in the hands (and name) of the master/mistress.

People who adopt a lifestyle obviously must work it around their everyday lives; though the relationship is in place all the time, its manifestations vary according to environment. Discretion is generally advised with regard to coworkers and other people not in the know, as well as young children. Coming out of this particular closet to family and vanilla friends takes quite a bit of tact and patience on both sides.

Unfortunately, a few people do demonstrate the wrong way to introduce loved ones to their lifestyle. Dan Savage once received a letter to his "Savage Love" sex advice column in which the sister of an apparently brand-new mistress wrote in asking for advice. The novice domme insisted on treating her slave like, well, a slave in front of everyone. This included people who were incredibly uncomfortable with the display, and she got offended if anyone called her out on it. Savage hit the nail right on the head when he responded, "Asking people to accept BDSM — the pastime, the lifestyle — doesn't give you the right to force other people to take part in it." (Savage, 2005)[4]

---

[4] By the way, this is good advice for anyone reading this, not just lifestylers.

Crossdressing

Crossdressing/transvestism is the act of dressing in the clothing of the opposite sex, either as a fetish or as a forced method of humiliation. It is not the same as transgenderism/ transsexuality, in which a person of one sex feels s/he has been born into the wrong body, and so dresses as the sex s/he identifies as in order to alleviate that dysphoria.

Male to female crossdressing is far more common than female to male. Part of this is because it's a lot more acceptable for, say, women to wear men's pants than for men to wear dresses. There's a strong element of humiliation for forced crossdressing, particularly for men, because for all the enlightenment that has been bestowed upon our culture, it's still taboo for "real" men to be feminine. Forced feminization in particular, therefore, may be an incredibly humiliating and submissive experience. On the other hand, it may also be a release for someone who is still in the process of resolving hir dysphoria but hasn't grown comfortable enough to explore it outside of a kinky setting. Forced crossdressing can manifest as torture, but it can also be an opportunity for a person to accept that s/he is dysphoric, and from there be able to do more work in addressing that dysphoria.

Crossdressing may not be that drastic, though. The aforementioned man-in-women's-panties may simply like the way the fabric feels, or may like being able to be a little femme. He may be entirely comfortable being male, yet enjoy a tangible way of getting in touch with his feminine side. Or he may have a fetishistic attachment to the panties themselves and view them as a sexual object (with or without another person wearing them). Crossdressing is also used in roleplay meant to play with the idea of gender—a lesbian who dresses to be her partner's leather daddy is a good example.

Narcissism

Anyone who has studied Greek mythology knows about Narcissus. So enamored was he of his reflection that he slowly pined away for want of himself and became a flower. (The Greeks seemed to be really fond of reverse anthropomorphization as a way to explain things.) The narcissism fetish involves becoming aroused by one's own reflection or image—self love at its most aesthetic. This may include having sex while looking at your reflection in a mirror, with your partner also focused on you, being aroused by trying on clothing and parading around in front of your own reflection, or even fantasizing about making love to yourself. It's not always the most discussed fetish, but it's going to play an important role later on in this book.

Object Fetishism

People fetishize all sorts of things. Body parts (feet are particularly well-known) are common, though certain parts are so widely fetishized as to no longer be considered kinky. Articles of clothing also may be fetish focuses, whether the fetishist is wearing them or not. Corsets are a particularly notorious fetish item; those who don't wear them love the look of them. Those who do wear them also enjoy the appearance, as well as the way it feels to have the body constricted and resculpted. Texture fetishists focus on the way a certain material, such as fur, leather, or vinyl feels. Potentially any object may be fetishized, though these are the more common ones. An actual person might also be fetishized, with the fetishist feeling a fascination that can only be expressed in having contact with that person.

Body Fluids

The three most common fluids that are fetishized are urine, feces, and blood. Urophilia includes golden showers and urine drinking, while coprophilia is attraction to fecal matter. Hematolagnia may include bloodletting, blood drinking, or arousal through the sight of blood on a person's body (or elsewhere). The blood may be venal, or, for some people, menstrual. The blood fetish may extend into a vampiric aesthetic, though this is far from universal in either blood fetishists or vampires (Kaldera, 2005, 83). Saliva, breast milk, and other fluids may also be fetishized, though are not as common, or at least not as well-represented.

Body Modification

While piercing, tattooing, and branding are increasingly popular forms of nonsexual body modification, they also comprise kink for some people. The pain of the procedure itself can be incredibly intense, moreso than standard whipping or flogging. In addition, the end results may be used to cement a relationship in a D/S or similar relationship. Some people also fetishize piercings, tattoos, and brands on other people.

Additionally, body modifications may be used to signify the relationship you have to your partner. For example, a submissive or slave who has made a lifetime commitment to hir dominant may get a tattoo or piercing signifying that bond.

Roleplay

Have you ever heard the innuendo laden one-liner, "Hey baby, let's play doctor"? That's just a very clichéd version of roleplay. A lot of roleplay fans enjoy the chance to pretend to be someone else, whether it's conqueror and captive, teacher and student, or pretending that one (or more, though not usually all) of the people playing are virgins again. Some folks even bring out elaborate costumes—ever wanted to be Catwoman seducing Batman (or Batgirl? Or both?)? Well, here's your chance!

However, roleplay can even involve invocation of deities and other entities. We'll touch on that a little later. Just be aware that roleplay is where you get to be—and play/fuck/etc.-- with anyone you can imagine.

We've only touched the tip of the iceberg; we'll go into more detail on the people involved in Chapter 5, and tools and toys in Chapter 6. Additionally, check out the bibliography and other recommended reading in the back of this book for even more relevant reading material.

Chapter Three: The Basics of Magic

Depending on who you talk to in the occult and/or pagan scene, the definition of what magic is will vary greatly. Although there may be a variety of ways to define magic, there's no right or wrong way to do it. In fact, the ultimate definition of magic could be argued to be, "Do whatever works, regardless of what that is." We don't endorse any particular style of magic over another, but rather would tell you that what's most important is that you discover on your own how and if magic fits into your life. Below are some definitions from different magicians:

"Magic is the manipulation of hidden forces or intelligences to produce a desired result [italics and bold are his]" (Black 2004, p. 20). This particular definition argues that magic involves working with spirits or otherworldly beings. By working with these beings, a person can shape and affect both hir internal and external realities.

"Magick is the science and art of causing Change to occur in conformity with Will [bold is his]" (Crowley 1994, p. 128). This rather vague definition is used by many occultists. The science can be thought of as the techniques, and the art as the innovation and creativity. Change is the desired reality a person wishes to bring forth, while Will is the unifying principle which unites the science and art together so that change can manifest.

"Magic is a set of techniques and approaches which can be used to extend the limits of Achievable Reality" (Hine 1995, p. 33). This particular quote complements a similar definition that Taylor has stated: Magic is the process of making possibilities into reality, and makes the improbable probable.

Magic can also be divided into subdivisions. Theurgy is magic that is focused on the worship of Deity (i.e. a god or goddess). The argument here is that Deity channels the magic and allows the worshippers to access it. Magic, in theurgical work, is religious. Thaumaturgy, on the other hand, is practical magic, with a focus on the scientific technique of magic (i.e. how it works). Here magic is invested in the individual as opposed to Deity (Bonewits 1989).

By now, you have an idea of some definitions of magic. There are more, but we'd have to write an entire book just on defining magic to do justice to all the definitions out there, not to mention all the various paradigms. What's important is that you make your own relationship with magic.[5]

Meditation and Gnosis

Meditation is one of the the primary methods of achieving an altered state of consciousness (ASC) in magic. Various cultures have different styles of meditation. In Eastern cultures, Taoist techniques focus on working with the internal energy of the body and strengthening the connection that energy has with the body (Chia 1984, Chia 2005, Chia & Abrams 1996, Chia & Winn 1984, Frantzis 2001a, Frantzis 2001b). Tantric and Tibetan meditations, on the other hand, focus on raising the energy of the body and pushing that energy upward to create mystical experiences for the practitioner (Feuerstein 1998, Lysebeth 1995). Yoga utilizes specific body postures that stimulate the hormones in the body and creates ASCs by retaining those postures.

In chaos magic, a western form of occultism developed in recent decades, there are two main divisions of meditation, excitatory and inhibitory. Excitatory meditation uses hyperstimulation in order to put a person into a meditative state (Carroll 1987). A person might dance until exhaustion puts hir into a trance. The auditory and vibratory stimulation of drumming can add to a trance dance, or may be used alone. Excitatory meditation also includes sex magic, where sex is used to create a state of mind (and/or raise energy) focused on a specific goal.

Inhibitory meditation focuses the person's awareness inward, while ignoring or detaching hirself from the sensations and experiences around hir (Carroll 1987). Taylor uses a meditation called "offnung" or open door (Ellwood 2005). In this meditation, he gradually relaxes his body more and more, drawing his consciousness inward so that eventually he loses awareness of all but what he's chosen to focus on.

Sensory deprivation tanks offer a similar experience, as can the application of blindfolds and earplugs, and even careful, almost

---

[5] For an excellent introduction to the different models and paradigms of magic that goes into much more detail than this, we highly recommend Nicholas Graham's *The Four Powers* (Immanion Press, 2006).

total immersion in a tub of water (with someone present to be sure you keep your nose and mouth above the surface). Kaldera has also used this technique. "Sensory Deprivation includes a wide category of activities, ranging from simple forms like blindfolds and earphones to complicated mummifications, enclosed tank systems, and more. By blocking out the world, the opportunity for bringing up wisdom from the depth of the soul through evocations is enabled" (2006, p. 61). He continues by explaining that this approach can also be used for possession work or for an awareness outside of the body (Kaldera 2006). The ASCs that are experienced can be very intense because the body is no longer distracting the mind with external stimuli. Sex magic can also involve inhibitory meditation, such as when the male makes no movement in the Tantric sex practices.

Once a person is exhausted and/or completely relaxed s/he is ready for gnosis, which is basically an intense single-pointed focus on the magical act at hand. For example, after a good scene and a rousing fuck, your mind may be the furthest away it'll ever be from the ESC. Use that moment to meditate or to focus on a practical issue you want to manifest, and you have achieved gnosis[6]. Gnosis can be best described as a state of knowing, within which changes can be made to a person's external behavior, as well as the internal issues associated with it. It is important to note that usually the internal reality that is "you" is inextricably linked to your part in the external situation manifested, and so the changes occur both microcosmically and macrocosmically. "As above, so below" also means "As within, so without," and what we do on one level of our existence affects other levels as well.

Invocation & Evocation

Invocation, in the traditional sense of the word, involves calling an entity and allowing it to interact with you and the world around you through the medium of your body. Invocations can involve full possession, such as occurs with the *loa* in Voodoo, but can also be much more mild, as in sharing the body with the consciousness of the god/entity present, with the magician retaining control and awareness of hir surroundings.

---

[6] We use the term "gnosis" as it is used in Chaos magic and more modern forms of occultism. The word is also used by ceremonial magicians to describe knowledge and conversation of the Holy Guardian Angel, as well as the enlightenment of Gnostics.

43

In *Pop Culture Magick*, Taylor offers a different take on invocation. He explains how to invoke yourself into a god, entity, or even another person (2004). This perspective argues that invocation is a two-way connection; if the entity can enter your body, you can also immerse yourself in the entity. The advantage of invoking yourself into an entity is that you can learn more about the entity and its influence, as well as create a more permanent connection with it. This approach can also be used between two or more people, and in that capacity, it creates very intimate connection.

Invocation doesn't have to involve any props or symbols, though some can be useful for making the magic more effective. Dressing in a particular costume or wearing an item you associate with the entity that you intend to invoke into you (or invoke yourself into) can make the invocation easier, as well as prove to be an effective form of banishing. When you take the item or costume off, the invocation symbolically ends, and so the connection is closed down (though you may also choose to perform a formal banishing at the end of the ritual). Chants and visualization can help the invocation process run smoothly and help end it as well. Taylor uses a short phrase from the Deharan paradigm (based on Storm Constantine's *Wraeththu* books) in some of his invocations, "Astale (name of entity)." The phrase sets up the invocation for him, putting him in the frame of mind necessary to achieve the magical working he has in mind. Sometimes a strong visualization of the intended entity is enough on its own. If you are very familiar with the entity and can visualize and feel its presence, you can call it to you silently and let it take over. The importance of these tools and practices is to signal to your mind to prepare for work with that particular entity.

Evocation is the opposite of invocation. Instead of allowing an entity to possess you, you manifest the entity externally to you. The traditional approach to evocation has involved summoning an entity, trapping it in a triangle or other shape and carefully wording a request that you force it to complete. The request can range from knowledge about a specific subject to having a particular task accomplished in a set amount of time.

Our approach to evocation, when it comes to entities, is different. We prefer to work *with* entities, and treat them with respect. This approach is more effective for the same reason that honey is preferable to vinegar. Generally speaking, we'll call on the entity and negotiate an offering in return for the completion of a task. Either party is able to make suggestions or refuse a particular offering or task. While we differ from traditional attitudes about evocation somewhat, we have found that this approach has worked well for us time and again.

You'll probably find some deities, spirits and other entities to be easier or more appropriate for invocation and evocation than others. The Service of Mankind Church, which specializes in worshipping aggressive Goddesses invoked through human women and served by (generally male) slaves, tends toward Kali in particular (Anonymous, date unknown). In *Dark Moon Rising*, Kaldera calls on everyone from Inanna and Ereshkigal to Baphomet and Babalon, and Aphrodite is even described as "a mean femme top" (Kaldera 2006, p. 417).

Evocation and invocation aren't limited to ancient demons from musty grimoires and pantheons from long-dead cultures. We have both worked successfully with pop culture entities created by contemporary culture. For example, Lupa has worked with San, the main character of the Japanese animation *Mononoke Hime/The Princess Mononoke* as a manifestation of the huntress archetype. She found that San is every bit as effective magically as Lupa's matron goddess, Artemis. One of Taylor's most successful healing rituals involved evoking the crew of *Cowboy Bebop* as representatives of the five modern Western elements.

Additionally, you can invoke or evoke different aspects of yourself. The basic concept is that we are all multifaceted beings who primarily use only our egos. Aspecting allows us to bring forth other personae on a conscious, controlled basis. Aspects can be evoked as well; Lupa once evoked a negative aspect of herself that no longer served any purpose, destroyed it, and reabsorbed its energy so she could create something new in herself to replace what had been taken out.

You may even create the entity yourself. Created entities, also known as servitors, may have a variety of purposes ranging from making the magician aware of opportunities to protecting hir from negative energy to reminding the magician, while driving, of the speed limit and where potential traffic problems are. We won't elaborate on it here, but Taylor's co-written book *Creating Magickal Entities* discusses the process of servitor creation in detail.

Evocation in particular doesn't even necessarily have to be limited to conscious beings. In *Space/Time Magic*, Taylor touched on the idea of using memory as an evocation tool. In this case, the idea is to evoke through your memory a past altered state of mind or sensation that you've experienced. You can use this to recall and relive a moment in the past, or re-experience a particular state of mind again. Your body retains the memory of that sensation and through evoking that memory, you can experience that moment once again.

One final note on invocation and evocation, specifically with regard to kink magic: entities have the right to consent as much as humans do, in our opinion. This ties back into our philosophy that it's better to work with rather than command entities. For one thing, it's difficult to invoke a being who doesn't want to be there — and it's not a really good idea, either! As for evocation, sure, you could evoke an entity to be a bottom for you in solitary kink magic (which we'll cover more in Chapter 11). However, if that entity doesn't want to participate, A) it'll probably end up sabotaging any working you were creating, and B) you'll have trouble evoking that entity, and possibly others, in the future. Magicians do get reputations among spiritual entities, and continually abusive magicians may find that fewer and fewer entities will willingly work with them (which is probably a good reason why so many traditional magicians were, at one time, required to *command* anything they worked with!). Remember that respect goes both ways and that treating an entity with respect will get you much more than you'll get by abusing it and forcing it to do something it doesn't want to do. We both know of at least one case where the magician used mainly force to make entities do what s/he wanted. That approach eventually backfired on hir, with unpleasant results.

Energy Work

The energy raised during sex (and other activities) can be directed toward a variety of purposes, including creating an ASC for the participant(s). Energy raised in this way is the combined energy of all the participants and can be very powerful when directed properly. We've used this abundant wellspring for practical magic purposes and for inward journeys.

You already are using energy every day. Your emotions (energy in motion) are part of that. When you direct an emotion at someone or something, that energy will have an effect on its target. Belief, similarly, is another form of energy. The faith and belief you invest in magic or a person or a deity is a form of energy. Energy work simply teaches you how to consciously manipulate it to accomplish a goal. Healing is a common use of energy work; Reiki (a type of healing energy) is a well-known example in the magical community. The goal with healing is to repair physical, emotional, and even psychological pain under the right circumstances.

However, energy work can also be used to harm a person. Some of the martial arts use energy work. A martial artist can turn hir attacker's energy against hir, or the martial artist can direct hir own energy in a purposeful assault on someone else. Energy may also be directed in other malignant forms, such as curses.

Psychic vampirism involves taking energy from another person for the purposes of maintaining one's own health. It's theorized that many cases of psychic vampirism are caused by an inability to process the normal range of energy humans need to survive. Unintentional psychic vampires are not aware they are feeding on people and don't have conscious control over their actions. Intentional psychic vampires are consciously aware of their need to feed and can to some extent control that need, but in the end must still feed off of people (Belanger 2004, Kaldera 2005). An ancient Chinese legend discusses how old men would try to find virgins and drain the youthful energy from them during sex as a way of regaining their lost youth (Chia 2005). Anyone can learn to manipulate energy, to include siphoning it from outside sources. Be aware that energetic feeding can be dangerous for the donor and even the person feeding on hir. Part of this is because when you take in someone else's energy, you're also absorbing any energetic toxins s/he may be harboring. Additionally, deep feeding, which establishes a particularly strong connection, may result in unwanted emotional attachments that are particularly difficult to deprogram (Belanger 2004, Kaldera 2005).

Regardless of what paradigm you use, once you get used to working with energy you can use it for pretty much anything you can think of.[7] However, we also want to emphasize that it is important to be careful with energy work, particularly in a sexual/kink context. Such settings are highly charged with intimacy and openness, and through energy work it's very easy to establish a connection that seems to be very deep. This occurs because of the energetic nature of emotions (energies in motion); the feeling of connection that occurs in energy work can feel similar to the kind of intimacy that occurs over time between people in love, or between good friends. Unfortunately, just as casual sex can be mistaken for love, so can energy work be mistaken for intimacy.

---

[7] Taylor goes into greater detail on energy work, including paradigms and techniques, in *Inner Alchemy*.

Even should such openness occur, be careful and consider whether the emotions experienced are really your emotions, or are feedback you are receiving from the connection. We recommend that this kind of working be done with people that you trust who can control their emotions and who you've known long enough that you have a good sense of your feelings about and for them. Remember as well that the communication you have with people will tell you a lot about how in touch they are with their emotions and how well they can focus those emotions. And make sure that all participants perform a banishing afterwards to release any leftover energetic influences that might cause problems down the line. In fact, since we're on the subject, let's talk about banishment and similar practices next.

Banishment, Protection, and Purification

Banishment dismisses any influences, spirits, or presences that are unhealthy or need to be removed as a part of "cleanup" once the magical working is finished. A traditional approach to banishment can involve physically cleaning the ritual space you use to do magic. You might sweep the floor, dust any furniture, and clean any surfaces with a cleaner, all with the goal of banishing anything that doesn't feel right to you. In fact, when you've cleaned your house you might notice that not only is your place less cluttered and dusty, but it probably feels better mentally and spiritually. This is because when we clean we focus on improving not just the physical environment, but also the spiritual environment.

Every day we do rituals that banish energy or presences that don't belong around us. Taylor does several Taoist meditations, which not only banish any unwanted energy but also raise protective energy. Lupa is a fan of the Gnostic Pentagram Ritual developed by Peter J. Carroll, which uses vocal intonations and vibrations to remove unwanted influences from her energy (Carroll 1992). And, of course, there's the classic Lesser Banishing Ritual of the Pentagram (LBRP), as well as both serious and humorous variants thereof (try typing "Lesser Elvis Banishing" into a search engine sometime).

Another approach to banishment is to detach yourself from expectations and from your surroundings. Banishment by detachment means that you free yourself from the meanings that you associate with your surroundings and objects. As an example, you've probably had to occasionally go through everything you own and get rid of some of it. Has there ever been an object that you were really attached to, but you knew you should get rid of? You probably associated special memories or another kind of value with the object, and found you couldn't bring yourself to dispose of it. If you were able to detach yourself from those associated meanings, you'd find that the object would become just an object, having no special significance to you. You can perform an effective banishment by detaching yourself from the meanings you associate with everything. When Taylor does this kind of detachment, he's found that everything in the room becomes grey and lifeless. The meaning has been sucked out of the environment, and the objects in it, and they no longer matter. This can be a useful form of detachment to learn when you want to discipline your mind to stay focused on a task. Overuse of it, of course, can lead to serious issues with social balance, but it works well as a temporary banishing technique. It also allows you to take the proverbial "two steps back" from a situation and really evaluate it without the emotional involvement that can cloud judgment.

Protection, in magic, involves protecting yourself from people, places, entities, and energies that are unhealthy for you. However, it can also include protecting you from yourself and the self-destructive tendencies and energies that often become an influential part of our culture. For protection, Taylor usually uses his Taoist meditations to circulate and raise the internal energy of the body. This not only filters any outside influences that could be harmful, it also stabilizes the internal reality, providing order and structure to his thoughts. Being consciously aware of our thoughts and actions is often the most proactive form of protection.

Grounding and centering are two key concepts in protection. Grounding involves returning to a more stable ESC. When you've had an intense BDSM scene or magic ritual, you've probably noticed how hungry or dehydrated you are after it ends. This is why food and drinks are often kept on hand for people involved in a ritual (or a scene). It gives each person a chance to ground hirself back into physical awareness through a mundane activity. Additionally, maintaining physical health keeps us grounded in our bodies; if we're comfortable in our fleshly forms, we're less likely to try escaping them, if only through being a little too "headspacey."

Centering focuses your awareness on yourself. When working with your own personal energy, you are placing yourself at the center of it, assessing its condition, and taking control of it and the influences upon it. Taylor's daily rituals, for example, allow him to get in touch with himself and at the same time remove influences that he feels would be detrimental to him to experience or work with.

Some people create a trilogy of grounding, centering, and shielding on a regular basis. Shielding is essentially manipulating your energy to prevent unwanted intrusions by outer influences. A person may ground to anchor hirself to the Earth, center to get the necessary focus on the energetic connection, and then use the energy to create a shield around hirself. Shields can take a variety of forms. Some people visualize a sphere all around them (the "holy hamster ball"), while others envision a tight wrap of energy close to their skin, sort of like energetic chain mail or armor.

Purification involves cleansing yourself. Just as you take a shower to wash off dirt and sweat, so too it's good to cleanse the psychic grime you've accumulated throughout your day. Through your interactions with other people and events, and even with yourself, you'll find that your energy gets clogged up. To avoid energetic blockages (which can lead to emotional stress and even physical illness), it's important to purify yourself. A central idea behind purification in ritual is that the act of purification shows your respect to who/whatever you are working with, by cleansing your energy and self of any potential distraction. At the same time, you are mentally, physically, and spiritually readying yourself to perform the work at hand. It can also be a daily practice in and of itself, a spiritual hygiene routine.

If the definitions of banishment, protection, and purification seem similar to you, it's because they are. You might wonder then why we use three terms for what seems to be one function. It's all about the context. If we use the word "protection," we are discussing how a person raises energy to create a sacred space or place protected from unwanted influences. When we "purify," we are ridding ourselves of accumulated energetic detritus and, in a ritual context, dedicating ourselves to the working at hand. At the end of the ritual when we "banish," we are releasing the energies from the actual working we've done and letting them depart to accomplish the task we've asked of them.

Sigils & The Alphabet of Desire

The word "sigil" can have different definitions. In medieval grimoires, it refers to the symbol or seal that represents an entity you are evoking or invoking. In contemporary occult semantics, a sigil is created by representing a desire through an abstract visual or auditory representation, a practice popularized by Austin Osman Spare. A common method is to write out your desire, remove certain letters (such as all repeated letters or all but the first letter of each word), and then create either a word or a picture out of the letters that remain. This creates an abstract symbol of the original desire. The sigil is then charged through a variety of other means, such as focusing the energy of sex on it, or putting it in a public place and using the attention it receives to empower it. A word sigil may also be chanted or otherwise spoken aloud.

At the same time, the practitioner is also seeking to imprint the sigil on hir subconscious mind while consciously forgetting about its meaning. This allows the subconscious to manifest the desire (through the magician's actions) into reality, without having the conscious mind sabotage the process through preconceived notions, doubts or second guessing. Some people will destroy the physical representations of the sigils, but others, such as Taylor, choose to keep them around. The advantage of destruction is that you no longer have it as a conscious reminder. On the other hand, keeping the physical embodiment of the sigil is useful as a discipline tool. It forces you to actively train yourself to disassociate meaning from a given object. Use whatever approach works best for you, but don't be afraid to switch your tactics as needed.

The Alphabet of Desire (AoD) was first devised by Austin Spare. It's similar to the sigil (in contemporary usage) in that it is a personal set of symbols devised by a person. Only the creator knows the meaning of those symbols (unless s/he tells someone else, of course). Unlike a sigil, however, the AoD is not discarded after one use. Instead, as with any alphabet, it can be used again and again, and is useful for creating specific correspondences in a personalized system of magic. We've used AoDs for a variety of purposes. Taylor has used his to create a system of correspondences with the neurotransmitters in his body, and if you'll recall from the first chapter Lupa utilized hers in the collar binding ritual.

Divination

When many people think of divination, they think of an old woman in a tent reading someone's fortune with an ancient tarot deck or tea leaves. While you can use divination to get an idea of what the future holds, it's even more effective for exploring present and past circumstances. In that capacity, we can divine patterns of behavior and activity and consequently determine the best action to take in meeting a particular situation.

When you use divination to look into the potential future, the problem that arises is that the very act of looking changes the perceived outcome. Perceiving the tarot spread (or other divinatory tool) causes a reaction which changes and affects the overall success of the outcome. In this way, divination becomes an enchantment, and the look into a possible outcome serves to create a momentum toward the manifestation of that outcome. In other words, you're creating and feeding a self-fulfilling prophecy. This is not necessarily bad, if the outcome is favorable — but if it isn't, you're just making a bad situation more likely to occur.

The main problem is the assumption that the result of the divination is a *definite future*. This is largely due to the fact that the majority of people have a linear concept of time, that there is only one past, present and future. Space/time is a lot more flexible than that, however. When we divine, we do so to explore a number of possibilities available to us. We then choose the one that is most beneficial to us, and work towards manifesting it.

Another example of the limitations of traditional divination is the belief that you should do a divination every time you want to cast a spell. This supposedly informs you as to whether now is the right time to work that magic, but again it limits you to one particular outcome. It would better serve the magician to be aware of why s/he wants to cast the spell, explore all the possibilities, and then spend time manifesting those that are most likely or advantageous[8].

Magic and Psychology

We aren't professional psychologists, but we want to note that there is a lot of literature focused on how to incorporate psychology into

---

[8] For a more detailed discussion of the issues with divination, please refer to Taylor's *Space/Time Magic*.

magical practice. We've used these techniques in our own work, which includes kink magic. We find that blending magical work with elements of psychotherapy is an effective method of working through psychological issues.

It's important to note that seeing a licensed psychotherapist is a good idea, and something that shouldn't be discounted. If you are already seeing one, continue to see hir; if you aren't (and have serious issues), thoroughly consider your options and visit one (or more – it can take a few tries to find the right therapist for you, just as with any relationship). Both of us have benefited from professional help, and although we handle our issues now through our own practices, the professional assistance helped lay the groundwork so that we could do that effectively.

One good example is neuro-linguistic programming (NLP): "NLP deals with the structure of human subjective experience; how we organize what we see, hear, and feel, and how we edit and filter the outside world through our senses. It also explores how we describe it in language and how we act, both intentionally and unintentionally, to produce results" (O'Connor & Seymour 2002, pp. 3-4). NLP is a way of understanding how people communicate with each other, and how you can communicate most effectively with anyone. NLP teaches you to adapt to the different communication styles that are available to you. For instance, you may find through your word choices that you rely on one of the five senses over the others. Adjectives that focus on sound will tell you that you are an auditory learner and express yourself in a similar way. Therefore, if someone else is more of a visual learner, then s/he may not understand you. This causes a communication breakdown. Learning to rephrase your sentences to account for other styles of learning also leads you to a different state of mind (oriented on the listener's personal learning style).

Modeling, one practice of NLP, involves studying or reading how a person communicates verbally and nonverbally, and adapting your communication style accordingly. You can then communicate with that person and even act like that person, if you so desire. Study how the person interacts with others, and then change your patterns of communication to hirs. Mimic hir actions, the particular way s/he phrases words, even hir accent. In short, become the person. Actors use this approach to get into character. It's also useful in invocation, because paying attention to particular details allows you to access the consciousness of another entity much more easily.

Anchoring is another NLP technique that involves associating a specific thought process or memory with a gesture. People have both positive and negative gestures. A slap for one person could be a negative anchor that recalls memories of abuse, while another person, with the right conditioning, could perceive it as a pleasurable sensation of affection. Even the context of when a gesture/anchor is used will determine if it's a positive or negative experience for a person.

Fortunately, anchors can be changed and even used to trigger and deal with traumatic issues. As an example, for Taylor, being slapped is a negative anchor, bringing back memories of childhood abuse. While he wouldn't seek such treatment in everyday life, in a scene slapping has helped him come to terms with those memories, move past them, and heal the painful feelings from that period of his life.

NLP is just one example of psychology that blends well with magic. People have used other systems, including (but not limited to) Leary's Eight Circuit Model of Consciousness, Lilly's metaprogramming, and Jungian archetypes. Do be aware that if you decide to use psychological techniques in your magic for reprogramming yourself, you may find yourself startled by the intense depth of feeling that you experience. We'll get into more of the nitty-gritty on this topic in Chapter 10.

Addressing Chemognosis

We're well aware of chemognosis, the use of external substances to achieve ASCs for magical purposes. In the context of kink magic, we don't recommend using drugs, as they can impair judgment and cause more harm than good. Because kink magic is such a physical form of magic, and because many drugs can alter your perception of the physical plane, it's not a good idea to add the two together. Additionally, kink magic already creates ASCs. Adding a less controllable factor, including the chemicals inherent in any drug, artificial or natural, can distort the experience and cause the drugged individual to lose *all* control, not just the perceived control exchanged in a scene. You can stop a scene if it gets bad; a bad trip, however, you must ride to the end.

There is also the question of legality of these substances, which needs to be considered; while some entheogens, such as salvia divinorum, are (at the time of this writing) legal and relatively easy to obtain, others like psilocybin and LSD are prohibited by federal law, at least in the United States. Additionally, some state or local laws prohibit the use of the federally legal entheogens.

Finally, drugs can sometimes become a crutch, preventing people from learning other methods of trance. While some drug shamans can trance out with other methods, too many people use drugs as an easy trip and never learn any other method. Unfortunately, that doesn't work with kink magic. The discipline and training involved in learning to achieve ASCs is more important than any high or trip you experience with drugs, and it *cannot be replaced by those substances*. We remind our readers that it is your responsibility and choice whether to utilize chemognosis in general, but we strongly suggest keeping it separate from your kink magic.

Chapter Four: Sex and Sex Magic

It may surprise you to learn that, as we mentioned earlier, some people don't consider BDSM and other forms of kink to be sex. There are those in healthy monogamous relationships who will scene with someone other than their significant others, and it's completely acceptable all around. There may be a lot of play, stimulation, grabbing of tender body parts, even butt plugs and other plastic penetration, but as long as nobody's flesh enters someone else's orifices, it's not considered sex — on a technicality.

We don't think of sex as strictly the penetrative or oral acts centered on the genitals, but as an act of the entire body and spirit. We have had wonderful sexual experiences, together and with others, that never involved a single act of flesh-to-flesh penetration. This is why kink appeals to us so much -- because it's focused on a variety of experiences that aren't restricted to a specific area of the body. This was what motivated us to combine kink with sex magic, in order to produce a system of sex magic that incorporated all the benefits of kink.

At the same time, we want to draw on the available resources on sex magic to show how to integrate available techniques into a kink magic context. We also want to highlight what we consider flaws in sex magic practices, flaws that need to be considered carefully in the context of kink or vanilla sex.

Putting the Sex Back Into Sex Magic

We can just hear the gasps now from some of the people picking up this book:

"Look at this! A book on SEX magic! Oooh, sex! I bet I can work some real magic with SEX!!! Hey, look at this — it's SEX magic! I wonder if they talk about Tantra — that's all about SEX!"

"Oh, my, GOD(s)! How obscene! They're talking about SEX! Honey, get the kids — we're leaving!"

The above theoretical reactions may seem rather silly, but they reflect two common attitudes toward sex that we've encountered frequently. We were both raised in mainstream American culture, which despite its sexual bravado is actually quite sex and body-phobic. Many Americans are taught from an early age, through church or family or peers, that sex is dirty. We're forced to cover every possible inch of skin unless we want to be seen as sexually alluring; even breastfeeding in public is decried because "it's a NIPPLE!" While some parents are pretty good about having The S-E-X Talk with their kids, it's a situation of such stress that parents often worry how to explain to their newly pubescent young what those birds and bees are up to. Others never get up the nerve to do so, and the progeny have to learn from other sources.

Chances are good that the kids already have a decent idea. Sex is a cultural taboo, and so children, delighting in the thrill of the forbidden, talk to each other in hushed whispers on the playground about things they may have heard from an older sibling, or seen alluded to on television, or viewed in a pilfered porn magazine from a parent's supposedly secret stash. Granted, not all the information is correct; some children may think that babies come from kissing, or through their belly buttons, or other things that in retrospect are silly (but we believed it wholeheartedly back then!). Still, depending on the environment and peers at hand, by the time the parents have the nerve to have The Talk, the recipients may already know what's coming.

Regardless of how we learn about sex, there's a forbidden quality that comes with it. Look at the media — sex is a way of getting trashy attention and shock value, or something we must protect our children from. Talking about sex with other human beings is often expressed in bragging to one's friends (if you're male), or in hushed whispers and giggles over the phone with your girl friends, if you're female (stereotypically speaking, of course). You may be fortunate, as we are, to have friends with whom you can talk about sex in a calm, frank manner. However, most people have trouble talking about sex, which has led to misunderstandings about basic sexual dynamics and the perpetuation of ridiculous myths.

This prudishness even extends to reputedly sex-positive subcultures. The pagan community is one example that we have experience with. While we've met sex-positive pagans, we've also met some who were anything but. This is incredibly surprising, considering that one of the central themes of Wicca, the largest neopagan religion, revolves around the sexual cycle of the Goddess and God (and, by extension, all of Life). Beltane is second only to

Samhain as the most popular Wiccan holiday (and also celebrated by many non-Wiccan pagans).

Yet the Great Rite has been tamed; rather than an actual coupling between the high priest and priestess of a coven, in many groups the priest simply dips the blade of the athame (sacred knife) into the chalice held by the priestess. Most modern books recommending the Great Rite nudge people towards the symbolic rather than literal interpretation. With the increase in "family-friendly" pagan gatherings, more and more festivals are requiring people to cover up, or have restrictions regarding making out in public where the kiddies might see. Don't blame the festival organizers—they're following the standards of the mainstream society, to which even subcultures must adhere to some extent.

This is understandable in many cases; we don't advocate the presence of minors during sex magic rituals, or pagan parents deflowering their pubescent daughters with wooden dildos, or people running around in the buff where non-pagans could easily see during festivals on public land. What confuses us is a member of one coven making snide remarks about how another coven is too sex positive, insinuating that their own group is too serious for that ("and wouldn't you rather join our group instead?"). Additionally, we've seen discussions online and elsewhere opining how BDSM and similar practices have no place in paganism.[9]

However, sex and sex magic (kinky, vanilla and otherwise) are a part of the magical and/or spiritual practices of many pagans and magicians alike. To divorce it from the community because it's "inappropriate" sets a dangerous precedent. What next? Portraying Aphrodite as an innocent, untouched maiden? Having the reborn God in Wicca come popping out of a cabbage at Yule? Yes, these are extreme examples. Yet recent attempts to ostracize the more sex-positive elements of the pagan community (as well as other "undesirables") in the name of putting forth a good image to the mainstream do disservice to the diversity of the community.

Face it—sex happens. It's not going away, no matter how much we try to hide it behind closed doors or lay it at the feet of trashy celebrities. The prudish attitude of some pagans only reflects the conditioning of society. A healthy attitude toward sex, however,

---

[9] http://www.witchvox.com/wren/wn_detaila.html?id=7893&offset=0 has a good example of this debate. An article on a pagan festival that mentioned BDSM-friendly attendees sparked a three-page debate on Wren's Nest; the arguments on both sides are pretty typical of what we've seen overall.

breaks down internal energetic and psychological barriers. Sexual education, both in its technicalities and its techniques, leads to better health on all levels. These in turn make for much better sex magic.

Before you embark on any sort of sex magic, kinky or otherwise, we recommend exploring your own feelings about sex in its many forms. What makes you uncomfortable? Why? Is there any practical reason to be uncomfortable? How much do you know about the sexual functions of your body? Pick up a few books on sexual health and technique; we highly recommend the works of Mantak Chia, detailed in the bibliography, as good places to start.

Polarity in Sex Magic

One issue that occurs with both Western and Eastern sex magic is the polarization of the sexes. This attitude toward the sexes can be found in nineteenth century occultism (and even further back), "One calls the forces positive and negative, and one rediscovers them in good and bad, emission and reception, life and death, idea and action, man and woman (positive and negative magnetic poles) in the material plane and, conversely the woman (active pole) and man (negative pole) in the mental plane" (Randolph 1988, p. 10). The division into polarity is often used as a way of explaining the unity found in sex magic. It is the union of opposites. Intriguingly, a necessary ingredient often cited for the efficacy of sex magic is *love*. We are inclined to agree that love, in sex magic, can be very important as an energizer, though you can perform sex magic without so close a bond. Whether the *polarity* is necessary is another subject, as the union of opposites is by its nature a negation of polarity and its necessity. We feel polarity has caused harm and misunderstanding precisely because it is primarily cultural, as opposed to biological.

Polarity may seem like an obvious part of the universe. Most of the animals we interact with on a daily basis, humans included, are divided primarily into male and female. We have day and night, hot and cold, aggressive and passive, and other dichotomies. These often get attached to particular sexes; in patriarchal societies, men are seen as strong, aggressive and positive, while women are given weak, passive, negative qualities (If you don't think it's negative to be seen as womanly, consider how a woman in men's pants is treated compared to a man in a dress, transgenderism notwith-standing.)

What we, the authors, perceive, however, is that the universe is made up of continuums, not dichotomies. Day fades into night via dusk, and back again through dawn. Cold doesn't become hot without going through cool and warm. Passive and aggressive are only words we use to describe certain behaviors of varying intensity that all people possess, regardless of biology. Numerous invertebrate (and a handful of vertebrate) animal species are either hermaphroditic or have the ability to change sex. Our practice of magic has led us to blur the lines even more and accept that duality is an artificial construct created by those too afraid to think outside of easy pigeonholes.

The cultures that most modern magicians come from emphasize the male penetrative aspect, rather than the concept of a devouring vagina, and so the exchange of power is subtly active from the beginning. Incorporation of the penetrative power structure is a staple of sex magic, even in modern texts. In *Shaping Formless Fire*, Stephen Mace states that "The difference between men and women — in both anatomy and quality of energy — is conspicuous. Men eject the quickening jolt, the surge of power, that animates the enterprise. Women provide the form that can thus be stirred to life" (2005, p. 72). Unfortunately, this statement suggests a lack of knowledge about the female anatomy. The majority of men are ignorant of the fact that women can actually ejaculate fluid as well, and as such, by his criteria, are capable of that same energetic jolt.

It's not unknown for a woman to be the active magical worker, even in sex magic. A female magician may also use her vagina to draw in a male magician's energy and work the necessary magic, rather than simply acting as a vessel for the magic *he* works. Rather than passively waiting for him to come, she can take the energy. In at least one case, a woman has actively vamped sexual energy from men, without their knowledge, and then directed that energy toward her own purposes (WitchWitch 2006). While we don't condone her ethical values (as we think using a person's energy without hir permission is harmful to the person) it does illustrate that a woman can be the active principle. Additionally, it's quite possible for a woman to direct her energy into a man (or anyone else, for that matter), who then acts as the receptacle. If she wants a traditional symbol for this practice, it's relatively easy to purchase a strap-on; however, women are quite capable of directing energy into another person with or without a phallic symbol.

Polarity automatically buys into an attitude common in both Western and Eastern sex magic texts: the idea that having a vagina makes a person automatically passive/receptive, whereas the penis endows one with active/projective energy. The stereotypical polarity not only thrusts people into limiting roles, but it also oftentimes relegates the biological woman to being a convenience rather than a participant in magic, a mere cauldron in which the male magician stirs the elixir of life. But in sex magic, polarity is not a biological fact. "Our physical gender does not determine the type or amount of energy we have access to, and does not determine the roles we must play in sex magic workings" (Williams 1990, p. 108). It's important to remember that our gender does not define our roles when it comes to magic. Instead, if sex is something that must be defined, let it be defined in a way that is helpful as opposed to harmful.

Western sex magic generally involves heterosexual intercourse, with the focus primarily on coitus. The climax of the magic is assumed to occur when the man ejaculates, regardless of whether the woman has an orgasm or not (And we don't care how good your magic is — there's no way to guarantee simultaneous orgasm!). In this model, the magic is not complete until there's sperm floating around in the mix. Additionally, the focus is on the energy raised when the man orgasms, while the woman is merely the container for this energy. The woman serves no purpose that another man, a blowup doll, or the male magician's own hand could not fulfill.

Part of the problem is the misunderstanding or downplay of the female[10] orgasm. In Lupa's experience, a clitoral orgasm is much stronger than a vaginal orgasm. This is a common, though not universal, trait among biological females. A woman's difficulty in obtaining clitoral orgasm during coitus is a distraction, supposedly not worthy of concern until the "real" ritual is over — if even then. We wonder how many women have never had a chance to discover the existence of the clitoral orgasm, because they end up with partners who can't give decent face or hand (or who focus too much on their own pleasure to try). Others may end up with

---

[10] Please understand that although we refer to a person with a vagina as "female" throughout this chapter, we are not ignoring the fact that there are people who are biologically female but who do not identify as female.

unsympathetic partners who might discourage masturbation in a relationship as a sign of a bad sex life[11].

The vaginal/uterine emphasis bolsters an unhealthy attitude — the idea that giving birth (literally or figuratively) is a woman's highest function. This strengthens the idea that effective sex magic can only come about through coitus, because only coitus involves reproduction. While symbolic reproduction can be useful in creating effective magic, it is not the do-all and end-all of sex magic. Otherwise, why would so many magicians of all sexes use masturbation to cast sigils? Yet, from Cerridwen's Cauldron to the Holy Grail to the ceremonial Cup, women are generally limited in symbolism only to their uteruses. The clitoris is left out in the cold.

This emphasis also puts pressure on men. The need to perform, to be hard in an instant, and ready to have sex (whether you want to or not) is something that men experience, yet is also frequently unnoted because of the supposed male privilege. Not all men are ripped and buff (an image portrayed as the ideal man), nor do all men have high sex drives. Sex is not the only thing on a man's mind. Yet, inevitably, men are accused of "thinking with their dicks," or portrayed as sex crazy idiots. This stereotype is very harmful to men, pressuring them to conform to these images while also shaming them for having a perfectly natural desire for sex.

The secret to breaking this dichotomy starts at the very source of our genitalia. Every human fetus starts as female. It is only after three months that some fetuses develop into males. This means that everyone's genitals start out from the same basic little buds of developing flesh. The penis and the clitoris are anatomically analogous to each other, as are the testes and ovaries (Fox Internet Services, 2006-A).

There is no biological truth to polarity; polarity is a cultural concept, with meanings assigned to it beyond the physical basics. It's true that the bio-males and bio-females have different physiological functions. The man can produce sperm and the woman can produce an ovum, but these functions are focused on the same goal, and are similar in terms of what occurs, i.e. the man's body produces sperm as part of procreation, just as the woman's body produces the ovum for procreation. The difference is that a

---

[11] Admittedly there are men who are told not to masturbate while in a relationship. In truth, masturbating is not necessarily a sign that the sex life is going bad, especially if the couple/etc. are having regular sex. Sometimes it's a nice experience in and of itself, with or without a partner present, and it's good for both your health and your sex drive.

woman can carry a baby to term in her body, and a man cannot -- but the woman still needs a man in order to produce the baby. Yet there is still no definitive polarity, because that difference relates to a *biological function* as opposed to something more meaningful.

If we associate polarity with human biology, we are ignoring the intersexed, the spiritually androgynous, the gay and lesbian community, the transgendered community, and the people who don't have the full biological capacity to produce sperm or ova or otherwise reproduce. Polarity becomes a confining system that ignores the inconvenient truth that biology is capable of more diversity than just the dualistic male and female ends of the spectrum. We can also point to other species for evidence that polarity is not a biological constant.

To emphasize, human association of polarity with biology is a result of cultural beliefs about biology, a human-centric perspective that does not consider the variety of biological diversity that exists. We associate certain "values" with polarity. Men are the active principle and women are the passive principle in sex for instance-- but is that a biological reality? It is not. It is a cultural definition and a shoddy one at that. It focuses on assigning attributes to these roles without providing any biological basis for these attributes. Unfortunately, this assignation of roles has been harmful to women precisely because it has tried to minimize them and control their capacity to enjoy sex. It harms men because it's helped to create a stereotype where men are sex hungry creatures that only think about having sex. It's also harmed any person whose gender falls outside the traditional heterosexual sex roles. We've noted with some dismay that the majority of books on sex magic don't, for instance, offer much to the gay and lesbian community on the topic.

Some people might point to energy work as part of biology and say that is where this concept of polarity and men being active and women being passive comes from. While energy is an intrinsic part of the human organism and part of the biology of a person (see Lipton 2005), any associations/meanings made about it are cultural. We need to examine those cultural assumptions and ask why they have been emphasized and who it benefits to emphasize those assumptions about sex, energy work, and polarity. In our own work with energy, we've yet to find that women are passive and men active. Just because a penis thrusts into a vagina does not make the male active. We've found that such "polarities" are switchable in sex magic, and that women can just as effectively be the active principle. Some men, including Taylor, prefer the woman to be the active principle, directing the energy and focusing it as she sees fit. That preference is both a personal turn-on, and a recognition that a woman is just as capable of performing magic (regardless of the difference in biology). There is no difference unless people *make* a distinction of difference. Any difference on the biological level is a difference of physiological function, but not a difference of polarity.

In our opinion, magical practice would benefit to do away with polarity and the duality it inspires. Sex can be active or passive for both participants; if it's good sex, does it really matter which partner is active or which is passive? By overthrowing reliance on polarity, we undo the cultural harm it causes to people--of any gender. That harm is demonstrated by the murder of transgendered people who refuse the gender role assigned by their genitals, and choose their own gender. The current cultural meme of polarity allows for only two genders. As magicians, we owe it to ourselves and to others to decline this perspective in our magical workings, as our adherence reinforces a dangerous cultural attitude of intolerance.

With recognition of the cultural values that have infiltrated our notions of sex and sex magic, we can free ourselves of those notions and recognize that polarity is entirely cultural, subconsciously infecting us with values that are oppressive, restricted, and ultimately useless to the process of sex magic. We can then accept that whether it's hetero, homo, or pan sexuality being explored, the meanings we assign ourselves, each other, and our behaviors are uniquely individual, a way of making the sex act more meaningful and intimate--a celebration of diversity, not a reinforcement of stale cultural norms.

The Power of the Female Orgasm

For many women, the clitoral orgasm closely mirrors the male orgasm -- the senses are overwhelmed, and vigorous pulsing occurs in the clitoris, usually accompanied by powerful vaginal contractions. Stimulating the clitoris, obviously, is a bit different than stimulating the penis, though there are some parallels.

While the clitoris is not large enough to penetrate any orifices (without the aid of hormonal treatments), the clitoris and penis are essentially the same organ exposed to different hormonal levels. Some women even ejaculate from quasi-prostate glands. This ejaculate is of a different composition than male ejaculate, but can be used similarly in magic.

Powerful vaginal orgasms do occur in women, though perhaps not as easily or as ubiquitously as the porn industry would have us believe. Some women can only have them in connection with clitoral orgasms; other women may need more stimulation than a few thrusts to make them happen. The G-spot, the area in the vaginal canal where the paraurethral glands may be stimulated, and allegedly the source of some vaginal orgasms, can't be reliably found in every woman every time.

The female orgasm is every bit as magically effective as the male orgasm. Both involve the expulsion of a large quantity of energy coupled, with a state of gnosis that lasts the duration of the orgasm, and often for a time before and afterwards. Both have physical residues that you can use to paint sigils, consecrate or charge magical items, or use as a sacrament.

Sex, Blood, and Female Ejaculate

The habit of ignoring female ejaculate echoes the lack of focus on the female orgasm. The paraurethral glands in a female body are essentially analogous to the prostate gland in the male body, and during orgasm can release fluid, though usually in nowhere near as exciting a fashion as in the rare porno female ejaculation (Fox Internet Services, 2006b). Just because lube doesn't stem solely from orgasm doesn't mean it's just a byproduct of sex. It may be used to create sigils, consecrate ritual tools, and everything else semen is used for, short of impregnating someone.

Stephen Mace, when speaking of sexual fluids in magic, mentions that both semen and the fluid from the vagina can be used as Eucharists. Men can take the Eucharist directly, but he recommends women soak the liquid up with a piece of bread (Mace 1998). The Eucharist can be eaten to reabsorb any energy (and proteins in the fluid).

Menstrual blood is another fluid created by the female sex organs that leaves the body through the vagina. In Lupa's experience, menstrual blood has an aggressive quality all its own. This is due in part to the purpose of menstruation in general. It is a way for the female body to rid itself of toxins, and therefore is a monthly renewal process. Many women feel awful during their menstrual periods, but once it's over, the body is relieved of unneeded detritus, on both physical and energetic levels. As such, a woman can use menstruation as a way of purifying not just the body, but also emotions, from the frustrations and negative influences she's experienced in the previous month. Lupa also uses the menstrual blood for cyclic magic. She has a small, round piece of coral she keeps in a red pouch that she dabs with a bit of her menstrual blood each month. The coral absorbs the energy of the blood and stores it away until she needs it for abundance magic or other cyclic magic (Lupa 2005).

For Lupa, menstruation is a time of great strength. She can feel the changes in her body; the cramps that usually accompany the cleansing process are a sign that everything is in working order, and act as a further source of energy. It's a reminder that she is alive and well, a symbol of vitality. Additionally, as we have chosen not to have children, it is a reminder of the freedom of that choice. We renew our commitment to each other during her menstruation — because she is often the dominant during this time of the month, she needs to be able to display her strength, and for Lupa, the time of cleansing and relieving her body and energy of toxins is a high point. It isn't that way for all women, many of whom find menstruation debilitating--but magicians work with what they can.

There's also the issue of breaking taboos in ritual. The strength of menstrual blood contradicts the idea of the vagina as a passive receptacle of magic. The history of men fearing menstrual blood carries its own power for effective magic. For millennia, menstruating women were off limits to men in many cultures; they were considered unclean, and the Judeo-Christian bible goes into great detail (particularly in the Old Testament) about what to do if a menstruating woman makes someone or something "unclean" by touching it. Another reason, perhaps, that menstrual blood is a powerful magical component is that male magicians cannot obtain it (unless they ask the right woman nicely).

This source of blood is more than just a hole for insertion of a penis. The symbolism of engulfing and devouring are powerful enough that a minor archetype, *Vagina Dentata* (toothed vagina) has arisen out of the fear of the vagina severing the penis. An example of this fear is seen in the anime *Wicked City*, where the protagonist narrowly escapes having his penis devoured by a woman's vagina. The woman then turns into a spider-woman hybrid, completing the image of a predator. Mythology plays upon this fear, rendering the woman an entity the male must conquer, rather than approach and appreciate as an equal.

Rather than focusing on antagonistic polarity, we've found we prefer to work together. Our combined effort creates stronger results, and reflects the equality we have at the very basis of our relationship, both as lovers and as magicians. In the end, the power of the orgasm, regardless of whether it's male or female, will still be a power that we can all work with equally.

Chaos Magic Approaches to Sex Magic

TOPY's *Thee Psychick Youth Manifesto* offers a chaos magic approach to sex magic. On the 23rd of each month, on the 23rd hour, members in TOPY will masturbate or perform some form of sexual act, then take the sexual fluids, along with some body hair, blood, tears, or something else from the body, and put it on a sigil. They use the fluids and the sex act to charge the sigil. The TOPY members then send the sigils into a TOPY temple and keep them safe. The idea is to use the fluids to put the energy of the sex act to work: "Psychick energy and sexual energy are different names for thee same source: by ridding ourselves ov restrictions and thee forms ov control which have been imposed upon us we can coum into our own on more planes than one" (Anonymous 1996). The sigils are fired (i.e. the "spell" is cast) afterwards, when the sigil is mailed off and forgotten.

Another chaos magic approach is to physically express the sigil in the sexual positions you use. This requires flexibility and comfort with your body, "It's not a bad idea to create for every 'sacred letter' an individual body posture or a finger symbol and 'pronounce' your wishes with the relevant movements" (Karika 2005, p. 44). The formation of the sigil through the position of the bodies takes the magic to a new level, where the very act of sex is the sigil, as opposed to just the charging of the sigil. The firing of the sigil is the moment of orgasm, followed by the forgetfulness found in snuggling and pillow talk; the very loss of the position after sex is a symbolic forgetting. This technique works well in sex magic, because it emphasizes collaboration between partners, as opposed to the primacy of one partner over another.

Sex Magic in Tantra

Tantra, which has increasingly become popular in the West, is another form of sex magic. Or is it? The original Tantric belief system is *not* focused on only sex magic, and considers it to be only one aspect among many. The Western view of tantra, or neotantra, as it's more accurately known, is wholly focused on sex magic. It has been covered extensively in other works, so we will not elaborate on it a great deal here[12].

In neotantra, the focus is often on pleasing the woman. "By a very ancient tradition, Tantric goddesses and their female assistants (Dakinis) were not only dominant figures, but their images also showed a slain, conquered, or dominated male in a submissive position" (Anonymous p. 7). The man is supposed to retain his semen and not ejaculate so that he can continue to make love to the woman until she is satisfied. In this approach the man is passive, while the woman is active: "During maithuna, if the male remains quite still to avoid ejaculation, the shakti is active and controls the evolution of the ritual...During intercourse it is the shakti who gathers the cosmic rhythms while the shiva becomes immersed in her own magnetic energy until he feeds the 'divine vibration'" (De Lyesbeth 1995, p. 250). This approach can work to prolong sexual intercourse, though, in our personal experience, we prefer sex where action comes from both partners. If such action is desired, it is possible to prolong sexual intercourse without having to take the tantric route.

The main problem with neotantra is that many versions of it focus on sex magic to the exclusion of any other tenets of Tantra. In some cases, BDSM is incorporated into the practice of neotantra, as is evident in the *Essemian Manifesto* of the Service of Mankind Church (SMC), where men are treated as slaves and women are dominant by default. In traditional Tantra this approach would be viewed as imbalanced; the SMC only focuses on Kali dancing on the corpse of her husband Shiva, while ignoring other cycles of Tantra that are equally important: "He [Shiva] manifests the absolute stillness; she [Shakti] expresses the unlimited potency of Power or Energy. Together they symbolize the play of life and death, creation and annihilation, emptiness and form, dynamism and stasis" (Feuerstein 1998, p. 82). In Tantra, the interplay of forces is one that recognizes the value of the other and knows that balance involves not just staying on one end of the cycle. Additionally, people involved in traditional Tantra criticize neotantrists as primarily concerned with sexual pleasure and narcissism, as opposed to spiritual enlightenment (Feuerstein 1998). With that said, it's

---

[12] We recommend Feuerstein's work, which is cited in our bibliography, along with Julius Evola's *The Yoga of Power: Tantra, Shakti and the Secret Way* (Inner Traditions, 1992) as excellent books which offer a good perspective on traditional Tantra.

important to recognize that neotantra may be the only version of Tantra that a Western person knows, at least initially. We recommend researching what Tantra is as compared to neotantra, so you can determine if either practice complements the kink magic you want to perform.

The yoga exercises for Tantra are beneficial to both men and women. These exercises strengthen the internal and external muscles around the genitals, while teaching the importance of subtle movements and rhythmic pacing through synchronized breathing. Learning to control the muscles leads to better sex and better health benefits. Breath control is also essential, because it can teach you how to draw on the natural energy in your body more effectively[13]. The sensuality that is advocated in neotantra can be very useful for becoming comfortable with both your own body and the body of your partner(s). Some of the breathing exercises found in Tantra are similar to approaches found in Taoist practice, but there is one key difference. Tantric energy work focuses on establishing a connection with the divine, while Taoist energy work focuses enhancing the natural health and abilities of the body. We turn to Taoist approaches now.

To Ejaculate or Not to Ejaculate?

Taoist sex magic is primarily concerned with retaining sexual energy through total body orgasm, as opposed to the ejaculatory orgasm, which wastes energy. The Taoist desires the whole body orgasm because it creates more energy, which s/he can transform into life energy and store in the body (Chia 2005). Both men and woman can use the breath and energy work exercises in Taoist manuals to strengthen their muscles and their ability to work energy. Taoism polarizes the sexuality of men and women, through yin and yang. Yin is the passive energy of the female, while yang is the active energy of the male. With this polarization, however, each person has both yin and yang. Sometimes women can have more yang than yin, and the opposite can be true with men.

Some schools of Taoism support the retention of semen, while others say that there is no harm in ejaculation. It is true that with both Tantra and Taoism, if the semen is retained a man can last

---

[13] *Urban Tantra: Sacred Sex for the Twenty-First Century*, by Barbara Carrellas, offers some excellent breathing exercises and intimacy exercises that we've found to be quite useful.

much longer and have what is termed valley or full body orgasms. These can at times be multiple orgasms, as opposed to the usually singular experience of one orgasm with ejaculation. Frater U.D. describes the experience of a whole body orgasm, "The contractions of the whole body orgasm are, however, almost continuous - like being 'electrified'- with occasional explosions of greater intensity. These explosions can take place in any part of the body" (2001, p. 136). The experience of a full body orgasm can be quite intense and useful for healing purposes in sex magic, as well as just gathering energy. In healing, the full body orgasm spreads the energy into the entire body, raising the level of health by continually cycling the energy. Storing the energy usually involves putting that energy into the belly where the lowest tan tien (energy center) is located (Chia & Winn 1984, Chia & Abrams 1996). This is the safest place to put the energy, and eventually it cycles back to the genitals, starting up the energetic cycle once again.

It's important to understand that energy work is an essential part of sex magic. When we talk about energy in this context, we define it as the life force of a person, that essence by which life exists and which is present in everything. Taoists consider sexual energy to be part of life energy, "Your sexual energy is dependent on three things: The abundance of your sexual hormones, the strength of your kidneys, and the circulation of your bioelectric energy or chi" (Chia & Abrams 1996, p.191). In Taoist texts, the primary focus is on the male as the energy worker, though the authors will point out that women can do these exercises as well. The focus is on men because of ejaculation and the idea that men will lose their energy if they ejaculate (Chia & Winn 1984, Chia & Winn 1996). Many exercises involving breathing and sensing energy movement have been developed, partially to help prevent the loss of energy, and partially to develop techniques to use the energy not lost through ejaculation. Williams offers a different perspective: "When we learn to live within the subtle body, we gain greater control over the physical one. That requires developing the ability to visualize and to sense the movement of energy. We practice controlling our breath, channeling energy within the subtle body, and releasing that energy to achieve an intended result" (1990, p. 16). We believe that comfort with the physical body leads to comfort with the subtle body. For those interested in reading more on energy work, we recommend the books referred here, as well as Taylor's *Inner Alchemy*.

The real questions are whether energy is truly lost when a male ejaculates, and whether ejaculation is really a form of orgasm.

A frequent problem in sex, for men, is premature ejaculation. Most men don't know about the fine muscle control they can develop around the genitals, or the health benefits of doing so. We think the loss of energy is associated with premature ejaculation, as usually once a man ejaculates it may take some time for him to get an erection again. Whether the man has truly lost energy is subject to debate. Ejaculation can cause you to feel tired, but can also make you feel energized.

Most people don't understand how the natural energy of the body ties to the act of sex. Sex is a directive and creative action that not only allows for the propagation of the species, but also acts as a muse for creativity. Sex can create ASCs, and this in turn allows you to interact with creative levels of consciousness you might otherwise not access easily. Sex also circulates your internal energy, which can rejuvenate you while also dissolving any blockages. With the blockages dissolved, you will feel more creative and open.

Finally, most people don't understand the dynamic role that breathing plays in sex and in overall health. In the U.S., people breathe shallowly, which is unhealthy. By not fully exercising your lungs you can miss out on the benefits that deep breathing can offer; this extends to sex, "Your breath is the gate through which you can gain control of your body. Breathing is both involuntary and voluntary. In other words, we breathe regularly without thinking about it, but we can also change the rhythm or depth of our breathing" (Chia & Abrams 1996, p. 33). There are different types of breathing in sex magic. Fast in and out breathing is pranayamic breathing, which you can use to raise kundalini energy. The problem is that fast breathing usually leads to ejaculation. Slow and deep breathing does help control ejaculation, though supplementing it with muscle control is also important.

Chia & Winn advocate breathing in which energy is directed up the spine and over the head and then down into the belly. The tip of the tongue needs to be on the roof of the mouth to complete the circuit. This is done to circulate the sexual energy into the organs and rest of the body, thereby strengthening and improving the mental and spiritual abilities of the practitioner. Chia and Winn argue that nutrients and hormones in semen come from the various internal organs and glands in the body, although there is no definitive proof of this. By withholding ejaculation, those nutrients can be kept for the body, prolonging life for the man (Chia & Winn 1984). It is true that semen is a rich source of protein, but the hormonal changes that sex causes remain for some time after sex has occurred. To get the full benefit of the hormones, it's necessary to prolong sex:

> A moderate amount of sex tends to repair hormonal disturbances, to reduce cholesterol and blood pressure levels. Sexual activity alters the body chemically. The reason this happens is because every gland in the body affects all the others. Thus when sex hormones are stimulated, it stimulates the hormones secreted by the other major glands. (Chia & Winn 1984, p. 26)

Obviously, if premature ejaculation occurs the benefits are not fully explored, but somewhat lengthy sex with ejaculation does not rule out getting these benefits, despite what Chia & Winn would argue. There is no proof that withholding ejaculation causes a person to live longer, and the muscle and breathing exercises can promote a healthy sex life for older men who continue to ejaculate.

Some Taoists actually argue the exact opposite, saying that retaining semen is unhealthy. "Some people currently teach others how to press acupuncture points to stop the leakage of semen. Those who learn these techniques often become impotent, but they are believed to have terminated the desire for sex through Tao...People who contaminate their blood by avoiding ejaculation usually become thin and their faces show a yellow cast" (Nan 1984, p. 89). It's possible, if these techniques aren't taught accurately, that harm could occur, not just because of the physical actions, but also because of divergence of energy from where it should go. Sometimes energy circulation can overload a person's body. Ejaculation, and its energetic equivalent, allow a person to vent the pressure and let some of the energy out.

Taoists aren't the only ones to weigh in on this particular debate. Frater U.D. argues that it doesn't matter if the physical essence is lost, so long as the spiritual energy is retained (2001). In Taylor's experience, this has been true, as it is possible to draw the life energy out of the semen and bring it back into the energetic cycle of the body. The energy is *your* energy, after all, and as such, you have control over it. Many people forget this or don't know it, which creates the subsequent loss of vitality. U.D. points out the following, "It is not the material loss of semen which is to be avoided-but rather that *the etheric energy contained in the semen must be kept, refined, and stored or transformed into magical success-energy*" (2001, p. 129). As long as a person is able to master hir energy, it is entirely possible to avoid any loss of energy at all, should ejaculation occur with orgasm.

Ejaculation itself is not orgasm. Ejaculation can occur *with* orgasm, but can also occur without it (Chia & Winn 1984, Chia & Abrams 1996, U.D. 2001, Williams 1990). It's possible to have multiple orgasms, even with ejaculation, if the male has control over the muscles necessary to achieve orgasm. It's possible to have multiple ejaculatory orgasms in one sex session, provided a person has control of the muscles and awareness of how to circulate energy. You don't even need to feel tired afterwards. Taylor, for instance, has experienced multiple ejaculatory orgasms in just one session of sex. This has occurred through learning to use breath and muscle work to hold back the orgasm, while at the same time directing energy into the prostate gland, heightening the pleasure experienced there. The release of ejaculation, when it occurs, pulls that energy into the entire body of the male, causing a valley orgasm, which can be multiple as long as the energy is circulated throughout the body. It is our experience that the male will not have the loss of energy and health, or fatigue, provided both partners do the energy work properly and in a balanced manner. As long as both partners cycle the energy between them, it does not have to be lost. Instead, you can express it in union with your partner, and use it to create an even closer connection of healing, intimacy, and love.

It's true that a person who ejaculates will be less likely to have sex later in the day than someone who holds back his semen. The person who has retained his semen hasn't expended it. A person who expends the semen causes the testes to manufacture more, which takes time, and when ejaculation occurs, the blood stored in the tissue drains; this also takes time to come back. However, a partner can be satisfied, even if ejaculation occurs, by taking the time to build up with foreplay and to circulate the energy so that the lovers achieve balance between them. When ejaculation does occur, it's still possible to have repeated sex. By learning techniques that help a man insert a soft or semi-erect penis into his lover, sex can occur again and still be good for both partners. Also, when you've ejaculated during sex and your partner is not completely satisfied, stay inside. Don't withdraw. The penis, even soft, can still bring your partner satisfaction. It isn't the penis itself which creates enjoyment as much as it is the manipulation of the breath and the muscles in the pelvis and stomach. If a man learns how to control the muscles and use subtle movements, he can bring a lot of pleasure to himself and his partner while doing very little.

Learning breathing and muscle control is worth the effort, as are learning how to experience an ejaculatory orgasm and a valley orgasm. Both types have their benefits. The valley orgasm is good for healing and storing energy, while the ejaculatory orgasm is excellent for directing energy toward a specific goal. In such cases, the fluid will retain the energy and you can use it as a sacrament for an object or for other purposes. Remember, in the end, your energy is your own and isn't something you have to give away through orgasm.

Most of the information available regarding ejaculation and energy concerns male ejaculation. It is a great disservice to the field of sexual knowledge that female ejaculation has, throughout history, been largely ignored. However, Lupa has found that both muscle control and proper breathing can also help those with female bodies to both improve orgasm and lengthen "staying power." Her experiences with the loss or retention of energy is that, regardless of which one she chooses, the end result is still an overall feeling of purification.

The Nitty-Gritty: Safe Sex, Partners, and Negotiation

Okay, lesson #1: we can't get you laid. That's up to you. We sell books, not playmates. However, that being said, here are some things to keep in mind about sex in a kink magic setting once you do have that special someone(s).

You've probably heard it a thousand times before, but here's a thousand and one: play it safe. If you have enough money to buy this book, you have enough money to buy a box of condoms and/or dental dams. You can also check your local Planned Parenthood about resources for free or cheap birth control and STD protection. If you enter "free condoms" into any search engine, you can find a number of sites that offer free samples of name brand condoms. (If you need a dental dam and all you can find are condoms, cut a condom from end to end and unroll it for an easy alternative. Just beware of bad-tasting lubricants!) As for manual sex play, rubber gloves are available in both latex and latex-free at any place that sells general health care items.

One of the first conversations you should have with someone that you're considering as a kink magic partner is the sexual history talk. Honesty is highly important when it comes to things like STDs and partners past or present. Insist on safe sex, too—yeah, condoms, dams and gloves are a pain to deal with, but they're still more fun than, say, herpes or gonorrhea.

Another important conversation is regarding personal limits. What is everyone comfortable with? What might be possible under certain circumstances? What's absolutely out of the question? This applies to kinky stuff as well as vanilla sex; there's a great checklist that includes just about everything at http://www.bdsm-education.com/checklist.html. We also suggest coming up with a safe word, safe action, or other way of letting everyone else know when enough is enough.

Finally, remember — there's no rush. A large part of successful sex — and magic — is rapport. Specifically with regard to kink magic, we encourage working with someone you already know, because the distraction of getting to know each other is already out of the way. However, if you're currently single, we don't recommend kink magic as a first date activity. It requires a solid connection among all participants, and we're not just saying this to be elitist. If you've ever had a one night stand, then compare the quality of casual sex to sex with someone you're more attached to and familiar with. Kink magic works better if you're able to concentrate on the matter at hand without worrying if someone you're creating magic with likes having their elbows nibbled or not, or if you're too concerned with trying not to laugh at a partner's melodramatic scening to pay attention to the pathworking you're supposed to be doing. And if the first few attempts at kink magic don't work out quite like you expected, just remember — if at first you don't succeed....[14]

In the meantime, check out Chapter 11, which is partly dedicated to the solitary kink magician.

Vanilla, Anyone?

As much as we like kink, sometimes it's nice to just take a break and have some plain vanilla sex. Kink is intense, and too much can lead to burnout (though everyone's threshold varies). Variety keeps things interesting, though, and occasionally we feel like vanilla is our kink, since it's somewhat unusual for us!

The other advantage to vanilla is that it's a good time for honing sexual techniques without worrying about the added dimension of kink. Having a varied repertoire is a definite asset in

---

[14] ...try sucking eggs (With apologies to Crowley and Ministry.)!

many peoples' little black books; it would be a letdown if you were flogged to the point of extreme arousal, and then your partner ended up being a lousy lover. Additionally, while we enjoy kink with each other quite a bit, occasionally we take lovers on the side who have no interest in anything other than vanilla.

Just as many people don't limit themselves to one type of magic, so do many folks diversify their sexual experiences. The more variety you have access to, the wider your possibilities will be, regardless of what area of life we're talking about.

A Note on Giving and Taking

Whether its vanilla sex or kink, there is one universal principle about sex that we want to remind readers of: What is given is a gift, and what is taken is a rape. Taking involves doing something against the will of the person, depriving that person or injuring that person in order to obtain a moment's pleasure (if it can be called that). You should never take/force yourself on someone else.

You cannot take what is given willingly, precisely because it is offered. That offering is a gift, sacred in its own right and to be honored for what it is. Honor the person who gives freely to you and the sex you enjoy will be that much better because each person is respected.

Final Thoughts

It's now time to turn the subject to kink magic. Our purpose in writing this chapter was to present some of the issues relevant to sex magic. Obviously, we haven't written an exhaustive treatise on the subject, but for people interested in sex magic without kink, we recommend reading some of the books we've cited here.

Chapter Five: Who's Who (and What's What) in Kink Magic?

Here's where we get into you and everybody else who's mixing up the fetishes and the esoterica. Part of this chapter involves defining terms we're going to be using; the rest of it involves a brief exploration of how sex and gender aren't limiting factors in kink magic. It's going to be heavier on BDSM than anything else, but a lot of the principles are universal among kink.

All the World's a Stage...

Kink magic is all about psychodrama, and the players within that context. Those familiar with BDSM will no doubt have heard the terms "dominant," "submissive," "top," and "bottom," but there are also some that we've coined ourselves. For sake of clarity, we're going to explain how we *personally* define these terms as we use them throughout the book. Also, for our convenience (and because W/we F/find W/writing L/like T/this E/exceptionally I/irritating) we're keeping all the labels lowercase.

Some terms arose directly out of BDSM. Dominant, submissive, slave, top, bottom, and switch are the most common. There can be some confusion as to the differences between dominants and tops, submissives and bottoms, submissives and slaves, and why a switch isn't just a thin tree branch used to administer a sharp sting to tender flesh. The following definitions are the ones we've agreed upon.

Dominant: Also dom, domme, domina, etc. In a lifestyle setting, this is the person in charge. The dominant's control may be very subtle, barely noticeable to any but the most attentive eye, or it may be overt. An example of subtle control is a dominant who requests his sub to do something, knowing all the while that the only answer the submissive will give is a yes. An example of overt control is a dominant explicitly telling the submissive to do a task. The degree of control varies as well; some dominants maintain absolute control over their submissives, while others allow the submissive to retain independence in many aspects of hir own life.

Submissive: In a lifestyle setting, this is the person who gives up hir power to the dominant. The submissive may maintain a very playful attitude (the "bratty" sub), or one of great subservience. Again, the amount of control can vary from an obsequious, tame sub who complies with all requests, to a challenging and wild sub, who occasionally tests the ability of the dominant to maintain power over hir.

Slave: This is a submissive who has given up essentially all control to the dominant (who, in this particular paradigm, may be referred to as the master/mistress). A slave may go so far as to live with hir master/mistress and perform housework. Slaves may also legally sign over all material possessions to their masters/mistresses, particularly in a long-term relationship, though this is not terribly common.

Top: This is a more situational term. A top is a person who takes control within a specific scene, but not necessarily all the time. The top may live an entirely vanilla (non-kinky) life otherwise, with or without hir play partner. The top can also be a submissive/slave who tops a dominant at the dominant's request.

Bottom: Like the top, the bottom is also situational, and the other traits defined above qualify here as well. Very generally speaking, the top is the person wielding the whip, while the bottom is on the receiving end. A dominant may bottom to hir submissive/slave in a scene if the dominant so desires.

Switch: A switch is a person who may take the dominant/top and/or submissive/bottom roles, depending on circumstances and agreed conditions. For instance, we both switch. We both top and bottom, depending on the scene, and our relationship is equally fluid.

Bottom Space: Also known as sub space. This "space" is actually an ASC that a bottom experiences when s/he is topped. This state of mind is often the desired experience for a bottom, and usually will find that bottom mostly helpless. Sometimes the bottom will be unable to move or react, overcome by the various sensations that s/he feels.

Top Space: Also known as dom space. This "space" is also an ASC, but one which the top experiences. Instead of being helpless, the top feels a hyper awareness of hir surroundings and how those surroundings can be used to impact the bottom. The top may also experience an exhilarated feeling of control and power that loosens any inhibitions the top has toward actually topping someone. However, once the scene is over, the top may actually feel more vulnerable than the bottom as s/he fully realizes what horrible things s/he did to the bottom. As an example, sometimes when Taylor tops Lupa, after the scene is finished he needs reassurance and comfort because although what he did was what she wanted to experience, remembering that experience and the pain Lupa felt makes Taylor feel guilty. This kind of experience is natural and doesn't make a person less of a top. In our opinion, in this situation the bottom is responsible for the safety and well-being of the top.

We also have a couple of terms that we use in our personal practice:

Hard Topping: This is what most people think of when they think of BDSM (even if they're vanilla). Imagine the top that grabs a flogger and starts whaling away on the poor, bound bottom. While hard topping can have a lot more finesse than that particular example, it's generally topping that involves giving pain and intimidation.

Soft Topping: Less common, soft topping is sensual and gentle. It may include sensation play, such as rubbing things like silk and fur over the skin, or it may involve solid emotional reassurance for the bottom. Any pain that is administered is done lightly and only as a counterpoint to the rest of the play.

Breaking: To break a bottom is to bring hir completely under the top's will within the span of a single scene. This does not refer to a situation in which the sub has already surrendered hir will, as in some slavery-based relationships. Rather, breaking is a form of psychological edgeplay (a.k.a., "mindfuck") in which the bottom is swiftly and violently reduced to a point of extreme vulnerability. Breaking may involve physical bondage and discipline, mental triggers, and even energy work to shatter the bottom's shields and boundaries and completely bend hir will to the top. Obviously, this is not a practice to be taken lightly, but it can be a highly effective way of reprogramming unwanted, deeply-ingrained behavior patterns and conditioning. **We strongly caution you to be exceedingly careful with breaking or being broken; this practice can cause psychological, energetic and even physical damage if done improperly. We believe it should only be undertaken with someone with whom you have a very close, trusting relationship and who knows you exceptionally well (and vice versa). It should be considered an *advanced* practice and is not intended for those new to kink magic!**

We're going to primarily use top and bottom as generic terms in scenes, as not everyone playing may actually be in a 24/7 lifestyle. Keep in mind, too, that all of the above definitions are generalizations; your mileage may vary.

So, Am I Doing It Right?

There's really no right or wrong way to be kinky. However, there are some misconceptions about kink — and the people in it — that haven't quite died out yet. Keep in mind that these are heavily influenced by our own experiences and biases, and so you may or may not agree.

--Those who are in a 24/7 BDSM lifestyle are more genuine than those who aren't.

While 24/7 lifestyles can be incredibly intense and offer a lot of experience, that doesn't mean that they're the truest form of BDSM. Some people prefer to leave their kink in the bedroom. Others dislike the idea of giving up (or taking another's) control in their everyday lives. Even among individual lifestyle setups, there's no single "right" way to do it, just as there's no template for the perfect vanilla relationship.

--You have to be involved with the scene to be able to learn about or practice kink, and if you haven't been involved for X number of years, you have no authority.

The formal community does serve a definite purpose. It gives people who may not be as confident in themselves a safe space in which to explore. It's also excellent for face-to-face networking and discussion with other people. Larger communities often provide seminars, events, and other resources, which are a big reason why more people today are comfortable being kinky. However, if you don't have access to a community, if you dislike your local scene (and it does happen), or simply don't feel any need to be in a community, you can still learn about and practice kink. We recommend finding people you can talk to about kink, and there are plenty of kinky folk who avoid the formal community. You can also supplement with books, many of which sceners have written, though we wouldn't recommend relying on them alone.

In addition, age doesn't necessarily mean experience (or intelligence). We've met people twice our age who've been involved for less time than we have. In addition, a person who only scenes once or twice a year, no matter how old or for how many years, is probably going to have less experience than someone who scenes every night. Take each person—yourself included—as an individual. Don't get stuck in comparing; let each be who s/he is without trying to assign your preconceived notions to hir. In addition, don't sweat it if you meet someone who's been involved longer than you have. It's not a competition, and, as with many things, everyone is a student and everyone is a teacher.

--Real dominants don't bottom. Real submissives don't top. Switches don't exist/aren't genuine.

It's our personal suggestion (not holy writ, mind you) that everyone should try playing both roles at some point, just to have firsthand experience of what hir partner(s) are going through. There are dominants who have the idea that their dominance will somehow shrink if they ever bottom to anyone. That's not true. No one can take your dominance from you. It may be difficult finding someone you're willing to be vulnerable for, but bottoming isn't going to automatically negate any abilities you have as a dominant. If anything, it'll give you some insight as to why your submissive enjoys the experience so much. Similarly, some submissives are afraid of taking over the reins, so to speak. Don't be. It may take you a while to get used to topping, but if all else fails, think of things you like having done to you—then do them to whoever you're topping.

If you do decide to switch roles, be sure you discuss everyone's limitations beforehand. What you like to inflict when topping may not be what you like to receive when bottoming.[15] If you're really averse to the idea of taking the other side, you may want to examine why it makes you uncomfortable; there may be some negative conditioning within that you weren't even aware of.

As for switches—hell yes, we exist! Choosing not to play one part all the time doesn't make you less legitimate. We have found that switching enhances our experience quite a bit, particularly with regard to kink magic. Even when we aren't engaged in kink magic, knowing that we can both switch can make for a refreshing and needed change of pace in our play. Still, if you find that you prefer to stay in one role or the other, there's nothing wrong with that, either.

--Everyone's a switch (polyamorous, pansexual, etc.); they just don't know it yet!

In spite of Appendix D, in which we extrapolate on the advantages we've found in being switchable in kink magic, there are people who are quite firmly one way or the other, conditioning be damned. And there's nothing wrong with that. It can be a bit more difficult, for example, for a top to have a purification process through kink magic, but with some creative applications of kink magic principles, just about anything is possible. Some people assume that anyone who hasn't switched hasn't found the right top/bottom or simply has something wrong with them. While we suggest that there may be psychological reasons for a person disliking one side or the other that could potentially be changed with time and effort, we're not under the illusion that this covers every dedicated dominant or submissive.

The same goes for monogamous people. For instance, we've met a few people in the very sex-positive subcultures of various flavors who, upon meeting new people, almost immediately gave the disclaimer that they "weren't poly." While it gained a few healthy laughs once everyone realized that there was nothing wrong with that, it indicated to us that some members of the poly community had been aggressive enough with them to prompt such an immediate reaction.

Pansexuality is another assumption. While Lupa is quite happily pansexual, Taylor tends primarily towards a heterosexual

---

[15] For an elaboration on the advantages of switching in kink magic, please see Appendix D.

sexual expression. He is open-minded; however, he has had people assume, in various situations, that he was "bi like the rest of us." While some folks are pansexual in their kink (to a certain point), for others only one particular sex will do. Never assume that someone is interested in you based solely on their sex. This is a good rule across the board, come to think of it! Of course, the topic of sexual orientation segues quite nicely into our next section, in which we address...

Ladies and Gentleman (and Transgendered and Intersexed and Genderqueers and Monogamists and Polyamorists and ...)!

Kink knows no boundaries as far as who may play with whom, and how. Earlier writings on BDSM tended to be male-dominant and female-submissive, but newer writings may allow for heterosexuality, homosexuality, bisexuality, pansexuality, transgenderism, and so forth. It's not surprising, given that kinky people tend to be pretty open-minded as a whole. (That and the modern BDSM community has a lot of reasons to thank gay Leathermen of the Old Guard!)

There is much confusion over the precise uses of "sex" and "gender". Our sex-phobic society is so scared of the very word that the less-scary gender has replaced it in common parlay. Yet sex, in its strictest sense, refers to what's between your legs, while gender comes from what's between your ears. In other words, sex is the actual physical genitals you possess, while gender is your mental concept of your sexuality. LaSara Firefox points out the following,

> Gender is a culture-specific, collective, subconscious set of agreements about how people of each sex are required to present themselves in order to be accepted. Gender is different than biological sex, or sexual orientation...Gender is a fluid concept, one that can change dramatically in a very short amount of time, on both the personal and cultural levels. (2005, p. 33).

Gender is much more malleable than people realize, and isn't limited to the set of genitals a person has between hir legs. Additionally, not everyone identifies with whatever hir body is. Some transgendered people prefer to not have corrective surgery done, for example.

One cultural concept that's done a lot of harm is the polarity we discussed in an earlier chapter. The idea of polarity in both sex and gender may seem to limit sex magic only to heterosexual intercourse, as men are viewed as the masculine/active principle, while women must be the feminine/passive ones. Yet there are plenty of masculine/active women and feminine/passive men, and as we have discussed, biology does not limit the roles one can take in sex magic in general. In fact, masculine and feminine are poor synonyms for active and passive simply because of the confusion with physical sexes.

If active and passive energies transcend the physical body and are dependent on who's inside the body, then it's perfectly acceptable for non-heterosexual couplings to produce effective sex magic of any type. The exact mechanics of the manner in which the physical ritual is consummated may be different, but there's absolutely no reason why gays and lesbians can't work the same rituals as heterosexuals. This doesn't mean that one has to be "the man" and one has to be "the woman"! A butch lesbian is not "the man," and a feminine gay man is not "the woman" in a relationship People of all sexes run the gamut of active and passive energies, as well as the continuum between masculine and feminine.

The same goes for bisexuals and pansexuals. The fluidity that allows for attraction to more than one sex can translate into one's energy patterns. While not all bisexuals and pansexuals behave differently depending on who their partner is, others do. In the event that a bisexual/pansexual person acts differently towards different sexes, it's often a reflection of the individual personality, not a strict, "When I am with a woman I am like a man, and when I am with a man I am like a woman," sort of situation. Lupa reacts according to the way her partner at the time is presenting hirself; if she happens to be with a very feminine person, she has a tendency to slide more towards the masculine end of her personality, and vice versa.

Transgendered people are another good example of breaking through traditional sex roles. A male-to-female transgendered person is not "a man in a dress." She is a woman, albeit one whose genetic structure does not match who she is as a person. Anyone who has known a transgendered person both before and after hir transition will notice that hir energy matches the gender s/he identifies with, regardless of what hir genitals indicate. Similarly, while some intersexed people (those born with genital features of both the male and female sexes) are content with the gender assigned to them at birth, others experience gender dysphoria. This is particularly exacerbated by the common practice of doctors "fixing" the genitals of an intersexed baby right after birth, usually by removing any male organs (which still doesn't account for male genetic material and hormones, which may play a key role in later development).

The recognition of androgyny is comparatively new within the arena of sex and gender identities. An androgyne is a person of any sex (not necessarily intersexed) who feels that s/he is a combination of male and female internally, or a completely different sex combining qualities of male and female. Both of us identify as androgyne despite our bodies. Lupa adds "genderfluid" to her qualifiers, given that she sometimes feels male, sometimes female, but generally somewhere in between, while Taylor tends to be more settled in the middle, identifying with neither gender, but instead incorporating aspects of both into his identity. We use the pronouns that match our bodies to help alleviate confusion, though we've been known to answer to the "wrong" words. Androgyny means that we embody both active and passive principles, as well as masculinity and femininity, and utilize whatever we need at any given time.

In the same way, traditional polarity can be completely shattered by polyamorous groups of three or more. Polyamory literally means "love of many", and is an alternative to monogamy that generally involve committed, long-term relationships (rather than short-term flings, as in swinging). Everyone in a polyamorous situation is aware of who's involved with whom, and there's a strong emphasis on responsibility both to the self and to all others involved. While not everybody in a polyamorous situation may be having relationships with each other (i.e., Person A is involved with Person B and Person C, but Person B and Person C want nothing to do with each other), polyamorous triads and other poly relationships can still work effective kink magic together. It might take a little bit of time to figure out the details of who's going to be doing what and when and with whom, but no more so than in a BDSM scene or non-sexual magical ritual.

What this all really boils down to is that anyone can perform kink magic whether you're a straight heterosexual monogamous couple, a butch/femme polyamorous lesbian pair seeking a third (and perhaps a fourth), or a pansexual transgendered triad. You can be hardcore dominant, submissive-only, or switch roles at the drop of a cane. There's a place for everyone here.

Chapter Six: Tools (and Toys) of the Trade

There's a wide selection of tools and toys for use in kink magic. Some of them overlap both kink and magic in vanilla ways, but just about anything in either area of practice may be adapted to the other. We've already covered some of the historical crossovers of kinky things and magic early on in the book, but here are some modern ideas on what's out there and how to incorporate it into kink magic.

Bondage Equipment

Bondage equipment consists of ropes, cuffs, handcuffs, chains, and other equipment used for the express purpose of physically restraining a person. When the bottom is restrained from moving, s/he can't escape or struggle against the top. The top can use bondage to emphasize the powerlessness of the bottom's position, or just to give the bottom a feeling of security in being bound (and therefore "kept" by the top). S/he can even use it for seemingly cruel humiliation. A fetish night that Lupa used to attend regularly was also attended by a couple who owned a wide variety of creative toys, including a little cage on wheels (human pull toy!) and a swing on a tripod (wind the sub up tight, then let hir go and spin until s/he gets sick!).

St. Andrew's crosses, spanking benches, catherine wheels, and other similar equipment are used to hold a person in place during a scene. The person can be suspended and in some cases moved around on devices that are better suited for play than the average bed. In fact, you can tie people to all sorts of interesting things; the aforementioned fetish night featured an old one-person kneeler from a church to which people could be bound in very interesting ways.

In magic, bondage equipment is not used as often, but it has its places. Probably the best known, albeit somewhat veiled, use is in British Traditional Wiccan initiation rites. According to Aidan Kelly, the binding of a probationer for initiation into a coven is most often to heighten the sexual tension. The procedure is drawn from the Masonic Cable Tow, a cord that binds an initiate and is used to lead him into the initiation ritual (Kelly 1991, p. 50). Magicians of various flavors may use bondage as a method of accessing ASCs through restriction of movement.

In kink magic, the bottom may be bound and contained for part or all of a ritual. This allows the top to contain and direct hir bottom's energy for a particular magical purpose. As an example, the top may bind the bottom in such a way that forces hir to look upon a sigil, and then, through pain and other stimuli, raise energy with which the bottom charges the sigil. Conversely, the top may simply draw energy out of the bound bottom and charge the sigil hirself, reducing the bottom to a convenient magical battery. Release from bondage may symbolize crossing a certain threshold into a new stage of life at the climax of initiations and other metamorphic magical applications.

Bondage may also heighten a guided journey or other transcendental experience. The state of helplessness that tight bondage can evoke may help to trigger an ASC; additionally, the stimulation of the skin via the bondage equipment can heighten the bottom's awareness of hir body. Sensory deprivation is a well-used technique for stilling and focusing the mind, sparking all sorts of interesting states of consciousness.

We find bondage gear especially useful for kink magic because it not only serves to physically restrain the bottom, but from a magical perspective, it can also bind and shape the person's will and energy toward a specific end. Make sure that the bondage equipment is comfortable and not too tight. You don't want body parts losing circulation and going numb (loss of circulation is physically dangerous). Ideally, you should be able to put two fingers between the skin and the gear, which allows enough movement to keep circulation going.

The bondage gear contains and binds the bottom's energy. The act of putting on cuffs, ropes, collars, leashes, etc., should be an act that emphasizes both the helplessness of the bottom and the realization that hir energy is the top's to use as s/he sees fit. When you put an anklet or wrist cuff on, for instance, tell the bottom that you are binding hir energy. When s/he sees the clasp closed and the buckle pulled tight, or the key put into the lock, s/he should feel as if s/he can no longer direct her energy. In fact, the equipment may be specifically charged prior to use for this very purpose.

Floggers and Other Implements of Pain

In kink, participants use floggers, riding crops, and paddles to inflict pain on the bottom (and occasionally on the top!). This can be a stimulus for pleasure or for punishment — or even both, as many people find different types or intensities of pain to be enjoyable or tortuous. For instance, a person who can tolerate only a light massage with a flogger may enjoy having dozens of sterile needles inserted under hir skin.

In modern magical practice, the best known example of pain infliction in magic is the initiation in Gardnerian Wicca and some of its derivatives. While not all covens *use* a scourge (small flogger), some still adhere to Gerald Gardner's inclusion of it. Kelly theorizes that the use of the tool was more sexual than is often claimed. According to him, the founder of Wicca was enough of a flogging fetishist that he may have required the flogging to become aroused enough to perform in the Great Rite (an act of sex magic symbolizing the unification of the Goddess and God) (Kelly 1991). This has been disputed as a personal attack (Frew), while others explain the flogging as merely a way to stimulate the blood flow and attain the necessary trance for ritual, and for overall purification. However, as Gardner has long since been deceased, there's really no way to know for sure what his actual purpose was.

Floggers and other implements in kink magic are used not only to inflict pain, but also to direct the energy of the bottom and deliberately induce ASCs. The sensations might be used to push the bottom into a divinatory trance, or as a way of directing the bottom's energy toward a practical purpose of magic. Floggers et. al. can also be used as wands, suitably, as wands are associated with air. Taylor uses the riding crop as a wand, directing Lupa's attention with it, and sometimes gathering the energy into it and then releasing it with a whip-crack motion.

Collars, Jewelry, and Other Marks of Ownership

Collars are often used in kink to denote the dominant's ownership of the submissive. Sometimes a leash is added as another way to reinforce the authority of the dominant. Jewelry can add a subtle touch, as in making the submissive wear a specific item every day, but without anyone else's awareness of the jewelry's purpose. For a long time, as a mark of his submission to Lupa, Taylor wore a red ribbon around his wrist. By wearing the ribbon, Taylor showed his full acceptance of Lupa's ownership.

Tattoos have similar uses. Because the tattoo is a permanent part of the body, a person should be careful about deciding whether s/he really wants it for the rest of hir life (or until s/he can either get it covered up or removed). If the relationship ends, the ink could be an uncomfortable reminder of the past relationship. As an example, we only got tattoos once we got married. For us, choosing to get married indicated a willingness on both of our parts to make a dedicated commitment to make the relationship work. We use the tattoos to remind us of that choice and the importance of honoring it and each other by making the relationship continue to work, even when it isn't easy. Marriage isn't always the best marker of commitment for everyone, however; some people are against the very idea, and as of this writing, the U.S. government is still incredibly closed-minded about gay marriage.

In magic, jewelry symbolizes or embodies various energies, influences and entities. Jewelry might be worn as a magical artifact for a specific purpose. Taylor made a black leather pouch that he wears as a reminder of the most important focus of his life. Generally, any jewelry worn will have private meanings for a magician, though more generic symbolism may be recognizable to other magical folk. For example, a person may wear a pentacle to signify to others that s/he is a Wiccan, but on a more private level, the necklace may have been a symbolic gift from a deity, or it may be charged with healing energy.

In kink magic, the submissive wears a collar that binds hir to the dominant. By wearing the collar, the submissive allows the dominant to not only own hir, but also to control and guide hir magic. The submissive can wear other jewelry that serves a similar function but is less shocking to the vanilla world. Tattoos are also used in dedicated relationships. The choice to accept the tattoo signifies the dedication of the submissive to lifelong service to the dominant. It should be noted that even though the submissive is bound to the dominant, the dominant is also connected to the submissive.

Knives & Pinwheels

Knives are used in both kink and magic, though for different specific purposes. Pinwheels are used only in kink. It's important to emphasize the need for safety in using these tools. Always sterilize your blades before and after play, and make sure they're sharp. Any area of the cut skin should be washed with a sterilizing agent such as rubbing alcohol or iodine. Anti-bacterial soap is also useful. Finally, have your first aid kit and adhesive bandages on hand for any messiness that may occur.

The threat of using a knife in a scene is, in some ways, more effective than actually using it. The sheer terror of the *possibility* of being cut and watching blood flow can be quite stimulating for a bottom. Taylor will sometimes trace the edge of the knife on Lupa's skin and then with a saliva-moistened finger, he'll touch the area where he "cut," telling her that she is bleeding. The threat of leaving a scar on the body is also useful, if the person is narcissistic.

The pinwheel is for sensation play, as opposed to cutting. The spokes can cut or puncture if enough force is used, but it's better to apply a light touch as even a slight amount of pain can send electric tingles through a person.

When knives are used in a magical context, they may be associated with the element of fire or air, depending on the tradition. Generally, the knives are not used to cut someone, as after such an act the blade would need to be purified and consecrated again. Knives are ceremonial tools, and give a symbolic representation a physical reality.

In kink magic, knives and pinwheels are used as tools to open a person up or cut away an impurity. Although these tools can be used as traditional athames or ritual daggers to create sacred space, we prefer to use our knives for opening up each others' energy or even as a tool to build trust.

Candles

Candles are popular in both kink and magic, though for different purposes. In kink, candles not only provide atmosphere and lighting, but serve as an instrument of fire in temperature play. One partner can sprinkle hot wax on the other, burning the skin just a little. For people with above average body heat, candles may not be appropriate to use, as the heat of the wax will hurt much more. In that case, we recommend using ice packs, which provide the sensation of cold. Using the sensation of cold on a person with high body heat still provides some painful stimulation, but the contrast of the cold also provides some relief. Likewise, if a person has a below average body temperature it's better to use candles than cold packs, because the heat provides a contrast to the usual sensation a person feels.

In magic, candles provide atmosphere and light, and may also serve ritual or magical purposes. The color of the candle may symbolize a particular meaning or be associated with a particular deity the magician is working with. Additionally, candles are used in practical magic. A magician may rub oils on the candle and burn it to manifest a specific purpose, or even carve a sigil in the candle, that charges the working as it burns down and fires it when the candle is completely gone.

In kink magic, the use of candles is combined for both of the purposes detailed above.

Body Paint

Body paint is an excellent way to get in touch with the sensuality of the body and can be very expressive. For kink purposes, we recommend paints that can be washed off easily with a shower and some soap. You can find body paint in costume shops, with a decent variety of colors, and acrylic paints are available in any craft store.

In kink, body paints are just another tool to mark the bottom, in whatever manner the top sees fit. Even things such as eyeliner and lipstick can be considered body paints, and are used to force feminize a person, embarrassing or humiliating hir by making hir into the opposite of how s/he thinks of hirself.

In magic, body paint is often used for invoking an entity or evoking a memory and/or issue. Body paints are symbolic representations of the invoked forces and sometimes even channel those forces for the person. They may also be used simply for decorative or celebratory purposes.

We've also used body paints to bring forth the pain of insecurities and then wash away or purify that pain. The paints symbolically represent the pain and the consequences of the painful experience, which hold us back.

Costumery/Ritual Garb

Costume play, or "cosplay" for short, comes from both kink and magic (as well as various unrelated subcultures). In kink, it is associated with roleplaying. A person may wear a costume and pretend to be someone else, such as a heroic knight or a savage barbarian. Such roleplaying can allow people to act out fantasies in specific settings and in specific ways. How believable those fantasies are is up to each person.

For magic, costumes become gateways for invocation, calling in a specific entity by dressing like that entity and adopting its mannerisms. Costumes can also be ritual garb worn for magical workings, such as wearing a specific color robe or costume that symbolizes a connection to the ritual you are performing.

In kink magic, the ritual wear varies depending on the mood of the people and the work being done. It enhances the setting and establishes a certain vibe or tension for the work.

Drums and Other Sounds

The sound of a drum or your favorite CD can be useful for creating an atmosphere and building up to a scene or sacred space. In kink, music is used to create a sense of ambiance. The music can be any kind you favor. In general, however, we've found that for us music is more of a distraction than a contributor to a scene, with rare exceptions; your mileage may vary, of course.

In magic, drums or music as background sound helps to focus a person on the tasks at hand. In a drum circle, the drums guide and move the dancers in a trance. In ritual, the drums may likewise create a trance state for participants. Music also creates atmosphere and a sense of space that isn't set in mundane reality. We rarely rely on music, because although it can be a useful aide for magical workings, it can also be a distraction. If you choose to use music, try ambient music that will become background noise for you.

In kink magic, the drumming can sometimes be background drumming. The top can drum on a bottom's body, creating a rhythmic smacking that puts the bottom into an ASC. The addition of pain provides an extra sensation that reinforces the rhythm and sounds of the smacking. It's important to occasionally alter the intensity of the blows, as much to not exceed a pain threshold (and thus potentially jar the person out of trance) as to guide the person through different parts of the journey. We rarely use this kind of working in kink magic ourselves, at least as a primary method of inducing ASCs, but it's certainly viable for those with the ability to endure long periods of pain.

Incense and Oils

Incense and oils can provide a nice touch to a scene, in terms of sensation play. The aroma can add to a specific atmosphere, and certain oils may feel wonderful on the skin (though beware of allergic reactions!). In magic, incense and oils usually have specific meanings associated with them, and the magician uses them in rituals to reinforce those meanings. Incense is particularly useful in evocation to provide, via the smoke, a substance that an entity can use to assume physical form. Oils provide scent and create associations.

In kink magic, incense or oils enhance the magical working and build up the sacred space. The top may have the bottom anoint hir with oil as an act of worship and devotion. Massage oils with a dash of a particular essential oil may also be used, through those with sensitive skin may want to test the oil to avoid whole-body irritation! Incense may be used as a way of focusing the bottom's mind on the current magical task by permeating hir sense of smell with a scent that is closely tied to the scene at hand.

Crystals and Stones

Crystals and stones generally aren't used in kink (other than, perhaps, decoration), if only because the damage they could ostensibly cause is much more permanent than a flogger, depending on the creative ways one might use them. In magic, though, crystals/stones serve a variety of purposes. Crystals placed on a person's body can align and heal the energetic body of the person. Stones can mark ritual boundaries for the participants. In some cases, stones have even been anointed with body fluids, such as the Lingam stones, for purposes of increasing the fertility of a person (Van Lyesbeth 1995). There are other uses for anointed stones, however, including using a stone with menstrual blood to help with cyclic magic (as described in Chapter 4).

In kink magic, crystals and stones serve similar purposes. You might anoint a stone with sexual fluids to increase fertility, or use the stone as a binding object for a bottom. Additionally, certain types of stones placed within the scene area can help enhance certain energies; as an example, amethyst might be used to enhance a scene meant to heal, or to add to a soft topping.

Energy Work

We covered energy work in an earlier section of this book, but it's worth noting as a tool in itself. While there is no physical form to energy, magicians rely on it frequently for a variety of purposes. They use energy for healing, for helping to open a person emotionally, for feeding or draining a person, for inflicting harm, and also for defense. And as always, the energy can simply be directed toward a specific function or purpose.

Mind Machines

Some tools can be useful aids in achieving ASCs and are generally not harmful to use, unless you happen to be epileptic. We emphasize that these tools should not take the place of the discipline and self-mastery of meditation, but we've found these tools to be useful in kink magic scenes. The mind machine is one such tool, and has several different makes and models.

Mind machines use audio strobe technologies to induce ASCs. Music or other sounds are heard through headphones and are translated into light pulses, which then flash onto your closed eyes via goggles equipped with strobe lights. The different sounds direct the different patterns of light, although you can adjust the intensity of the strobe lights[16], dimming them or brightening them as needed. This is especially useful if you want to overload your senses and put yourself into an excitatory state. Adjustment of the volume of sound can also be useful for inducing a similar state.

There are a number of models of the mind machine available on the market, though we are familiar with two in particular. Depending on your funds and your preferences, you may wish to obtain only one model or both. The Proteus model is a model which allows you to program different sounds into your mind machine, so that you can make your own soundscapes. This is highly useful for those who are musically inclined. With a CD player, the Proteus can play audiotech CDs, which are CDs with specific sound frequencies built into them that the strobe lights respond to. The downside to the Proteus is that it doesn't have some of the features the Sirius model has. The Proteus model costs approximately two hundred U.S. dollars.

---

[16] Obviously if you have epilepsy or are otherwise prone to seizures, you should avoid this particular tool.

The Sirius mind machine doesn't have the Proteus' capacity for downloading programs that you create. However, it has enough other features to counter the Proteus, and it's cheaper, costing only one hundred U.S. dollars. While it can process the sound frequencies of the Audiotech CDs, it can also process the sounds of other CDs, so that if you want to use your mind machine for a ritual and really want to include your favorite Coil album, you can actually do it with the Sirius model – something you can't do with the Proteus model. Another feature is a built-in microphone that you can take to concerts, or to a location outside with natural sounds that you feel might be useful to experience as light sensations.

In the end, you have to decide which is most useful for you and within your price range. Consider the potential experiments you'd like to do with such technology. The magical benefit of using this machine is that it can be used to access different states of mind/gnosis, and as a way of achieving sensory overload. Other benefits include using it to help you sleep better, have more vivid dreams, and even help you study better or enhance your creativity and visualization skills. The last two skills are particularly useful for magicians, but all of the benefits can be helpful. With that said, you can also eventually get the same benefits through disciplined meditation. Balance using the machine with meditation and you should be fine.

Knowing When To Use Toys in a Scene

It's beneficial, in our experience, to keep the use of different toys to a minimum in any given session; for example, we may use the flogger for some scenes, but not every one. This creates anticipation and tension for the bottom, who will never be quite sure what toys will be pulled out *this* time. When a favorite toy is used, the bottom is surprised. At last, the bottom receives the sensation s/he wanted, but because the wait has been long and the sensation is unexpected, s/he is also shocked.

Shock is one of the most useful tools a top has. Unpredictability and avoiding routine will greatly aid the quality of the bottom's experience. For example, both of us like soft topping, but occasionally use it to induce a sense of security (which can then be used to the top's advantage!). A long massage, soft sensations, combing the hair, a build up of pleasure that can be extremely intense and then -- a hard smack from the paddle or flogger startles the bottom, throwing hir into a deeper subspace.

At least in some cases, this is true. For some bottoms, the sudden change in sensation may send them right out of subspace and into an unpleasant awakening. There's no single right way to use these tools, and you're going to have to play with each one to determine what works best (oh, the horrors of research!). Having a good variety to work with keeps the bottom from getting bored, and gives even more opportunity for exploration and experience.

We touched on safe sex back in Chapter 4; however, there are more safety concerns to address than avoiding accidental pregnancy and STDs. Before we go leaping off into a ten-hour kinky ritual with eleven floggers, three St. Andrew's Crosses, two extra slaves, and a ponyboy in a pear tree, let's take a moment to discuss some issues that may not be as fun, but are important nonetheless. We promise there'll be more play a little later, but we want to go ahead and cover this ground first.

Taylor has had seven near death experiences. His sixth one came about because he chose to work with a magician that he knew was not completely up front about the purpose of the ritual (Taylor knew this through prior experience). This magician's choice to be dishonest violated Taylor's consent, but Taylor violated the "safe and sane" principles by choosing to work with someone he knew wasn't trustworthy. The other magician also violated the "safe" principle because he exposed Taylor to the risk of serious health issues (overdose, allergic reactions) by dosing him with an unknown entheogen (without Taylor's specific agreement or consent). By not telling Taylor about the entheogen, the magician violated the trust given him. The shock of experiencing something that he wasn't prepared for put Taylor into a near death state. Ironically, Taylor likely would have agreed to the ritual if the magician had simply been honest with him from the start.

There's a great deal of responsibility in both magic and kink. Both are practices that can seriously harm you and/or other participants, and the consequences can include anything from permanent physical injury (or in rare cases, death) to long term psychological imbalances. None of these are conducive to healthy sexual and/or magical relationships.

In the above example, some of the responsibility was on Taylor. He chose to work with someone he didn't trust completely and the consequences that unfolded were not good for him. But some of the responsibility was also on the magician who chose to put Taylor into a dangerous situation without fully informing him of that fact.

Kink and magic share the risk factor, especially when other people are involved. Both leave participants vulnerable on a number of levels. They may be opening themselves up energetically, psychologically and otherwise to new influences and states of consciousness that they may not be ready to handle. Old wounds and sensitive areas of the psyche may trigger entirely by accident. While most people would think that kink is more potentially physically hazardous, we've heard enough stories about wayward blades, flammable ritual garb too near the candles, and people tripping over random objects on the floor during ritual to realize that vanilla magic can have its share of dangers, too.

Both SSC (Safe, Sane and Consensual) and RACK (Risk-Aware Consensual Kink) originated in the BDSM community. The acronyms stand for essential elements of play, but again apply to magical practice as well. Since SSC is the older and (at this point) better-known of the two phrases, we'll start with it.

SSC

First off, let's talk about safety. You are responsible for your own safety. This includes assessing whether you feel comfortable working with someone. If you feel even a slight discomfort with another person, don't work with hir. You will be doing everyone a favor by declining. Trust your instincts and intuition regarding people you might work with. Remember, you are responsible for yourself and the consequences of your choices. This extends to the effect you have on others; when you opt to play with someone, you can't blame your actions on your partner(s). If you end up cutting someone else a little too deeply, your first action shouldn't be to hastily throw on your clothing and bolt out the door, tossing a quick, "I'm sorry," over your shoulder. You'd better be releasing the person from whatever bondage s/he's in, cleaning the wound and, if necessary, getting hir to the hospital for professional patching up.

Be aware of your limitations, physically and otherwise, and make sure those you play with are aware as well. Endorphins released by pain can cause you to tolerate more damage than you realize you're receiving. In cases of bondage, check extremities to be sure blood is still circulating. If they're tingling, going numb, or turning red or white, remove the bondage equipment immediately. The same goes for excruciating pain or muscle cramps. Certain toys, such as clamps, should only be applied for a few minutes at a time anyway, particularly to very sensitive areas of flesh (and ideally, should be adjustable). Take people's individual health issues into consideration, too. That person with respiratory problems probably shouldn't be subjected to any sort of asphyxiation play, and someone with a bad back may want to be careful when flogging a partner—you don't realize just how much you use your back until you injure it and then try to move around as usual!

Specifically with regard to flogging and other percussive pain, it's important to know where you can strike the body, as not just any part will do. For instance, striking the lower back can hit the kidneys or other internal organs, while the neck is full of all sorts of sensitive areas like the spine and throat. Any blows to the head, even slaps to the face, should be done with extreme caution; if you hit someone on the ear just the right way you can damage hir ear drum. Make sure you know what parts of the body are safe to hit, and be sensitive as well to each bottom's individual safe areas.

Just as you wouldn't play or scene with a person you don't trust, it's not a good idea to practice magic with just anyone. Magic is similar to BDSM in the sense that you are opening yourself to the people you are with, and vice versa, and it can be easy for an unscrupulous person to take advantage. Your partner could siphon off energy without your consent, or evoke an unwanted entity or energy into you. Even if the person doesn't go to these extremes, if you don't trust someone, that distrust taints the magical working and can cause the magic to fail, or to work in a manner that's detrimental to everyone involved. Similarly, scening with someone you don't fully trust can hamper communication and result in someone getting hurt. Either way, negative experiences can ruin whatever relationships (and reputations) might have been involved.

Sometimes emergencies do happen. It's a good idea to learn first aid and CPR, and keep a fully stocked first aid kit nearby. Make sure there's a fully functional phone at the scene; if it's a cell, make sure its battery is fully charged. In case something happens, be sure that anyone bound or otherwise restricted can easily free themselves or reach help, and that they are not dependent only on you for that help (what if *you* are injured and they are trapped in restraints?). Lastly, if you're in a scene and a serious injury occurs, call 911 and get to a hospital. You may have to answer some awkward questions, but better that than a serious injury becoming a fatal one.

There are several questions you can ask yourself to gauge the sanity of a situation. What are the potential risks involved in a scene you're planning? Addressing safety concerns should help to curb some of the more obvious potential dangers. As we mentioned above, be realistic about your limitations and those of others. An hour of spanking may sound fun in fantasy, but if the most you've ever gotten were a few quick whacks on the butt with a fly swatter, you may want to reconsider. Sometimes it's a matter of not overextending yourself. If you've only recently discovered magic and have read maybe a book or two, and someone offers you a chance to lead a group of other novices in an intense Underworld journeying meditation to meet a deity you've never heard of, it's probably a good idea to pass.

Speaking of other people, is everyone involved considerate of each other's feelings and limitations? Unfortunately, in both kink and magic, there are a lot of flakes who will believe anything they are told — and then spread it around like authorities. There are also predators who are out for a fix for their self-esteem and who will feed off of anyone they can. Flakes and predators can be subtle. If you've been around the block a few times, so to speak, you get a pretty good idea of how to tell the good ones from the bad ones. However, even seasoned pros can occasionally be fooled by someone with tons of charisma, or who is careful to keep hir public reputation safe. It may take a while for the shine to wear off and the decay underneath to show, by which point the flake or predator may have yet another victim.

The best thing to do is just talk to the person. Talking avoids falling prey to the gossip of others. Both the kink realm and the pagan and occult communities are riddled with politics and drama—just like any other group of people—and it's easy to get suck(er)ed into it without even trying. Make it a policy to take people as individuals and judge for yourself, but also balance that with advice from people you know and trust. Be wary of the new acquaintance who tries to manipulate you into hir own end of the political spectrum by badmouthing a whole string of people without any provocation. Your best bet is to just take everyone with a grain of salt at first, and see where your trust lies after a time.

"Consensual" involves honesty. Be honest with each person you work with. If you intend to do magic with a person, but don't tell hir what you're doing, you're breaking hir trust. When we say to be honest, we don't mean that you have to explain in excruciating detail what will happen every moment of the ritual/scene. But everyone should have a general idea of what will happen and what hir role is. You don't want to surprise someone, or worse, have hir find out later that you had an ulterior purpose for the ritual you did with hir. Not only is this manipulative and unethical, but it taints the magic. Likewise, you should work with people who are upfront at the beginning about what they expect from you and what will happen.

Honesty also applies to the BDSM scene. Be honest about your past experiences, or lack thereof, what you want and/or are willing to experience, and any health-based limitations. If something occurs in a scene that makes you feel uncomfortable (in a bad way), stop the scene and communicate with everyone involved. Communication will not only give you the much needed comfort and security, it can also prevent potential problems down the line. Moreover, it builds up trust between play partners, which is essential for having a healthy scene and relationship.

As a personal example, whenever we play with each other, if one of us calls the safe word, or the top simply recognizes that the bottom is in a state of mind that isn't healthy, the play stops. The top holds and talks to the bottom until s/he feels safe enough to either resume play (if so desired) or stop entirely and move onto other activities. We make sure to communicate and listen to each other, so that neither person comes away from the scene feeling harmed or ignored. Instead, resolution occurs and both of us feel secure in continuing to play with each other.

RACK

RACK is a newer acronym. Some consider it a "grown-up" version of SSC. One of the criticisms of the latter term is that it is too limiting. Gary Switch, who claims to be the originator of the term, says that, "If we want to limit BDSM to what's safe, we can't do anything more extreme than flogging somebody with a wet noodle."[17] He goes on to emphasize the self-responsibility and the edgeplay possibilities that SSC may sometimes seem to disallow.

RACK does have a different flavor than SSC. Take "Risk-Aware," for one thing. It differs from "Safe" in that it's willing to experiment, having done the research. Indeed, we need to be quite aware of the risks involved, as discussed above. However, how much risk is too much? For some people, knifeplay may be too risky because of the chance of an accidental amputation. However, others may love that sort of thing and get off on the very chance of that occurring.

Risk-Aware also emphasizes education and understanding of a particular topic. In the case of magic, there are magicians and

---

[17] http://www.vancouverleather.com/bdsm/ssc_rack.html

pagans too terrified of stepping outside of the safe parameters of their pet paradigm to try anything new. A good example of this is the fluffier flavor of Wiccan who is so stuck on the Rede ("An it harm none, do what you will") that s/he decries any practice outside of hir definition of "harm none." However, there are also plenty of magic-workers who play with "left hand path" magic, who summon Goetic demons, or who (gasp!) mix paradigms, pantheons and pop culture in wild magical experiments designed to shatter preconceived notions. These people tend to be aware of the risks, and proceed with self-responsibility and foresight. Were they to remain perfectly safe, they might even have stayed within the well-defined boundaries of an organized religion, rather than participating in the self-driven, self-liable practice of magic.

Consensual is one aspect that RACK shares with SSC, and we've already pretty much covered its importance above. Kink is also something that we're already familiar with. However, it brings the acronym a little closer to home (Switch explained partly for an aesthetically pleasing acronym, and partly because the vagueness of the application of SSC could theoretically — and humorously — lead to musings on "Safe, Sane, and Consensual trout fishing").[18]

Hurting Vs. Harming

It's all fun and games 'til somebody gets hurt, right?

The uneducated outside observer might get the idea that kink is all about hurting each other, so why would we even care about first aid? More is better, right?

Of course, we all know better than that. We often differentiate between *hurting* someone in the context of a scene, and actually *harming* them. Hurting someone includes, for example, a solid whipping to the point of safe word usage, or leading them through a very scary, but very effective, mindfuck that heals them in the process. Harming a person, on the other hand, includes pushing someone beyond their consensual physical and psychological limitations, either accidentally or purposely. You aren't an uber-dom/me if your greatest achievement includes putting a sub or slave in the hospital with broken limbs and massive internal bleeding. (If that is the case, we hope you're reading this from the safety of a prison cell.)

---

[18] http://www.vancouverleather.com/bdsm/ssc_rack.html

In the context of BDSM, hurting is pain that someone has consented to feeling. Hurting is okay pain, because although pain is experienced, it's pain that is used to enhance an experience, or open up a person. The pain is not intended to deliberately cause harm. Magic can also be painful; some magicians utilize their own blood in certain rituals, and may cut themselves to obtain it (though sterile lancets are a relatively painless alternative if only a small amount of blood is needed). Others may subject themselves to fasting, outdoor vigils exposed to the elements, or other tests of physical endurance that can bring discomfort in varying levels.

Harm, on the other hand, is the deliberate and malicious infliction of damage on a person. It is where the boundary between consent and non-consent is crossed. Harm can be physical, such as continuing to smack someone on the ass after the safe word is called, or it can be psychological, e.g. choosing to actually leave a person at a scene and go down to the nearest bar for a drink (and can also be physical if the person is bound) instead of only pretending to leave, but coming right back. In a magical context, harm can occur when one person feeds off of another's energy without consent, for example. When a person is harmed, it can take a long time for trust to be rebuilt.

The first time we presented a workshop on kink magic, one of the participants told us about a rather extreme mistress/slave situation. The slave did housework for his mistress as a part of his servitude to her. One day he apparently did the laundry incorrectly (maybe tossing a red sock into the white laundry?). His mistress punished him severely, to the point where she broke his arm. While we know that some people have serious pain limits, we've yet to hear of anyone who would consider a broken bone to be hurt rather than harm.

Avoiding harm can be done by adopting either SSC, RACK, or both, and then applying those principles. Of course, everyone's limitations are different, but communication is key. Another important tool in avoiding harm is the safe word/action.

Safe Words/Actions and Other Safeguards

A safe word (or action) is a common part of BDSM and is anything designated to communicate when a participant has had enough in a scene. While words are the most common, you can also select a safe action, particularly if someone can't speak because they've got a mouthful of ball gag. Additionally, some people may become so overwhelmed by the experience that they have trouble speaking, and so an action may be better.

The clichéd safe words are *red, yellow,* and *green,* in honor of that communicator of directions, the traffic light. Red means stopping an action right now, while yellow signals to take it slow and easy — red may be imminent if we keep going this way. Green, of course, means go, and more, and maybe even harder and faster.

Any participant may use safe words/actions at any time s/he feels it necessary. This goes for tops and dominants as well as bottoms and submissives. However, it's also a good idea for the dominant/top to periodically check in with the submissive/bottom, particularly if they haven't learned each other's body language and expressions yet. Any time a participant seems to be distressed, checking on hir may be warranted.

We occasionally encounter the opinion that real BDSM practitioners don't need safe words, and that a true dominant/top knows exactly how much the submissive/bottom can take. We respectfully, but strongly, disagree. The safe word/action is a safeguard that allows hir to notify the top when s/he's had enough (and vice versa, as we've mentioned). Going beyond that point violates trust and consent. If the bottom has no way of communicating this, then there's a real danger of injury, physical and otherwise. Less recognized, but no less important, is the top's need for the safe word/action. Top space is equally vulnerable, albeit in a different manner, and the top has the right to say "no." Therefore, we highly recommend having a safe word or action in place, just in case.

On the other hand, the safe word/action does not replace paying attention to your partner! This is a large part of why we emphasize our preference for playing with people we know well. It reduces the chances of problems occurring and increases trust and stability in the scene/ritual. However, it doesn't matter how well you know your partner — you can play with someone 999 times, and on the 1000th scene something could go horribly wrong. Therefore, we maintain that a safe word/action should be employed along with paying close attention to everyone involved. Even if it never gets used, it's better than having a situation where someone needs to stop, but the play goes on.

We understand that some people's edgeplay does involve pushing beyond the safe word. However, it's a good idea to talk about it afterwards to make sure that it didn't go too far. This means knowing your limits and everyone else's, which leads us to…

Know Thyselves (And Thy Partners)

Another theme that we've touched on both in this chapter and elsewhere is working with someone you know rather than, say, a one-night stand. Obviously, who you play with and/or work magic with is your own business. However, we're going to lay out our reasons for this particular preference right now.

Casual vanilla sex is risky to begin with. Anyone can claim to be disease free, spouse free, child free, and so forth. A fake I.D. (or no I.D. at all) can land you in bed with someone you could have sworn was of a legal age—until angry parents start asking questions about that little "oops" from a broken condom. And this isn't even including the low self-esteem that sometimes accompanies and fuels an unhealthy string of one night stands.

But those are all normal risks. We've been there, done that, had the quick flings and the worried ponderings. We've also had the thrill of a spontaneous encounter with someone that we might never get to sleep with again, the pleasant surprise of having that one amazing night with someone we initially found unimpressive, and the benefit of getting a completely different perspective on the joys of sex.

The problem with kink and the one night stand, or other encounter with someone that you really aren't that open with, is that the chances for disaster are increased. After all, allowing someone that you've never met to tie you up and beat on you is pretty crazy outside of a kinky context—and unfortunately even within the community there are people who are more predator than partner. Alternately, you take chances as a top, too. If you leave bruises on someone, and s/he decides afterward that it wasn't such a good idea, what's stopping hir from accusing you of assault? With the bias against kink that mainstream society still has, especially with regard to the law, you probably won't have much of a chance to defend yourself, SSC/RACK or not.

Additionally, someone who doesn't know you won't be as adept at poking around in your psyche. Someone you picked up a few hours ago probably won't have a very thorough understanding of what makes you tick—or how to put you back together if something goes wrong. S/he also won't have the amount of commitment that a good friend or long-term romantic/sexual partner has, and therefore, the chances of hir freaking out and running if something goes wrong are greater.

"But what about professional dominants?" you may be thinking. Well, sure, they definitely know what they're doing, and can top someone they've never even met before without a single problem. But note the word "professional." Not only do these folks have tons of experience, but the majority of them have been thoroughly trained to be good dominants. We'll also admit that there are people who have been in the Scene (or at least scening) for long enough that they've got an excellent eye for what their partners want, and have very thorough insights from their years of experience.

We're willing to bet that a lot of experienced kinky people aren't going to do much heavy scening with someone they just met thirty minutes ago. And we're not just talking about kink here; adding that extra dimension of magic makes it an even more potent experience. If you'll notice, most public pagan and other magical rituals aren't particularly intense. They're primarily celebratory, and often follow some formula that will be agreeable to the majority of attendees. The more intense, gritty workings are reserved for private settings, either alone or with people who know each other well.

You can certainly try doing a heavy pathworking with someone you just picked up from a fetish party. However, the chances of success will be a lot greater if you wait until you've gotten to know the person well in a number of settings, and are comfortable talking to hir about some of your most private secrets and stories — and vice versa. This means that you'll be in tune with each other, and will be able to tell more easily what needs work, what triggers and buttons are off limits, and what's likely to get the best response.

There will always be the exceptions to the rules. There's nothing wrong with that; both of us have scened pretty intensely with people we had just met, though magic wasn't involved. In the end, the decision is yours. However, this is why we take this particular stance in both our own lives and our writing. As with anything we present in a book or article, it's your prerogative to alter it to fit your own reality.

It Goes Both Ways (And We're Not Just Talking Bisexuality!)

A lot of this chapter has dealt with what to look for in partners for kink magic. However, it's a good idea to be the kind of partner you'd want to play with. This doesn't mean assuming that the other person(s) will automatically enjoy receiving whatever it is you like having done to you, or giving you what you enjoy doing to others. Rather, think of how you prefer to be treated.

Do you want respect and consideration? Good. You deserve it. However, you also owe the other person(s) that same respect and consideration. Think of it this way: you are exchanging valuable gifts of trust and openness when you work kink, magic, or kink magic with another person (among other activities). This gift can be incredibly difficult for some people to give, and if it's rejected or mistreated, it can cause trust issues to arise (or, for that matter, return).

This goes for people who've been together for a long time, too. It's easy to become complacent in a long term relationship; we start taking our partners for granted and start making assumptions on their behalf. This can lead to rude awakenings when it turns out that important things have been left out of crucial discussions.

Awareness of Psychological Triggers

Everyone has psychological triggers that touch off certain reactions and patterns. While these aren't physical tools, they can be used quite effectively on people. However, if anyone in the scene is unprepared for handling psychological triggers, the fun can quickly turn into a situation that no one wants. The less you know someone, the more likely it is you may accidentally set off a trigger you didn't realize was there (hence our warnings in the previous section). We offer the following thoughts on dealing with psychological triggers.

Be careful when poking around your or another's psyche. Much of our work involves delving deep into ourselves, which can end up bringing up personal demons and issues. Reenacting a rape from long ago for your very first scene is probably a bad idea, as is evoking Choronzon (a demon/entity that embodies the destruction that leads to rebirth) for a first-time ritual. We highly recommend working through a book such as Robert Anton Wilson's *Prometheus Rising* or Christopher Hyatt's *Undoing Yourself,* which are specifically designed as introductions to tinkering with your psyche, before working kink magic of this nature.

Also, let it be said now that *the psychological aspects of kink magic are not substitutes for professional psychological and psychiatric help!* Don't read this book and then go throw out your anti-psychotics and tell your shrink to go to hell. Also, it's not a good idea to mix alcohol and other mind-altering drugs with your kink magic. This includes prescription drugs; consult your psychiatrist about any possible side effects of drugs you may be prescribed combined with the intense experiences that kink magic may produce. (Sure, it's probably not going to be easy to tell hir that you're into kink, but depending on what medications you're taking, it may not be a good idea to expose yourself to things like mindfuck or severe D/S play.) Make sure anyone you're scening with also knows about the prescriptions you might be taking. Additionally, regardless of whether you're on psychotropics or not, don't stop seeing your therapist because you think this book can solve all your problems. That's not what we're here for.

If you have emotional issues, working kink magic with a trusted partner can be helpful in exploring some of the depths, but at the same time, it can also be a frightening experience. Worse, your partner may not know how to react to a situation in which you break down. We have had several experiences where the emotional triggers we hit released memories about prior abuse. While we were able to deal with those memories and come to a sense of closure with them, after hours of talking back and forth, it was not a fun experience. If you have *any* doubts, don't do a scene that hits those triggers. Wait until you are mentally and emotionally ready. Most of all, be forgiving of yourself. No matter how harsh the memories are, don't punish yourself for the past.

Communication, Communication, Communication

We can't stress the importance of communication enough (in case the header didn't tip you off). Before the ritual, as we've emphasized before, make sure that everyone's limitations are out in the open. Then construct a plan of what the ritual will involve. What's the purpose of the ritual? How many people will be participating, and how well do they know each other?[19] What elements of both kink and magic will be included?

During the ritual, speak up if you feel uncomfortable in a bad way. Use your safe word/action to stop the scene, and then be clear about what it is that's bothering you. If that entails continuing to

---

[19] For a couple of great books on pagan/occult group dynamics in general, we highly recommend Nick Farrell's *Gathering the Magic: Creating 21st Century Esoteric Groups* (Immanion Press/Megalithica Books, 2007) and Lisa McSherry's *Magickal Connections: Creating a Lasting and Healthy Spiritual Group* (New Page Books, 2007).

refer to "Master/Mistress" rather than "John/Mary," that's okay— it's better than being afraid to speak up because you don't want to offend. This goes for the top as well; check on the bottom if you have any doubt that there might be trouble, or if hir opening has opened *you* up to something you weren't ready for. An understanding partner/playmate won't complain about how you wrecked the scene if you stopped it because you were getting into the wrong kind of headspace, or because your hands went numb from too-tight cuffs.

Afterwards, talk about what happened. What did everyone involved enjoy? What wasn't so great? How is everyone doing mentally, emotionally, energetically and physically? Does anyone need to ground (return to an ESC)? Is there somebody who got upset and needs to talk it out? Again, don't be too afraid—or too proud—to speak up if you're not entirely happy with how something went. By communicating this with your partner(s), you can work to make the next time even better.

When Things Get Out of Hand

First things first—we can't address every possible disaster that might conceivably happen. (Our imaginations are good, but not that good!) However, we did want to address the more likely possibilities and what you can do to alleviate those problems.

Physical injury is a big one. If someone ends up harmed, stop the scene and remove any and all bondage. If it's just a small cut or abrasion, clean it and dress it, and keep an eye on it. In the event that the injury isn't something that you can treat with a first aid kit, get to a hospital as soon as possible. The same goes for injuries that don't heal at a normal rate, or get worse. This is a big category, but we trust you to use your common sense, especially in the case of things like compound fractures or two-inch-deep accidental knife gashes. Call 911 (or whatever your local emergency number happens to be) if the injured person is unconscious or otherwise immobile, or if a vehicle and driver aren't immediately available.

Psychological injury is another thing entirely. This isn't a matter of just slapping a bandage on an ouchie until it goes away. If you tweak your psyche the wrong way, it can have long-term effects. Again, this is why we stress knowing the triggers and sensitivities of all participants to the greatest extent possible. The more you know, the less likely somebody will hit something unexpected.

Again, in the event of an emergency, stop the scene and release anyone who's bound. Chances are good that the affected person will be crying, screaming or otherwise quite obviously upset. Some people go very, very quiet and unresponsive instead. Either way, if the safe word/action is used, or somebody just doesn't seem "right", it's time to pause what's going on and find out if there's a problem.

We've had a couple of situations like these ourselves. We've found that what works best is talking. The unaffected partner starts talking to the other, reassuring hir, touching hir gently if it's allowable (or giving plenty of space if need be). Under no circumstances will this partner get angry or yell at the upset partner. Patience is the most important component; the affected person is never forced to talk. Once s/he's ready, though, there's always an ear to listen and a shoulder to cry on, even if it's days after the scene and we're still working out the issue.

This is what has worked for us, and we've never had to do anything more drastic. We have exceptionally healthy communication that goes a long way in aiding us in, well, everything, kink magic related and otherwise. However, that doesn't mean that there isn't potential for worse issues. If talking still isn't helping after several hours, or the affected person seems to be getting worse or goes entirely unresponsive (or very loud and uncooperative) it's time to call for help. Try calling a crisis hotline and have the person talk to whoever's on the other end of the line. If this still doesn't work, it may be time to hit the emergency room again. In the worst-case scenario, go to the nearest emergency room; if they don't have facilities for psychological problems they can help you find a hospital that does. Bad ideas in this situation would include giving the affected person alcohol, or any drugs not already prescribed and scheduled.

Even if the affected partner does calm down to the point of functionality, s/he may still need quite a bit of aftercare (we'll talk more about this in a minute). Other people involved should be open to listening and helping hir deal with the situation to the best of hir abilities. However, if the situation just keeps getting worse, it may be a good idea to bring in a therapist (preferably kink-friendly if you can find one). This goes for everyone—it can be incredibly stressful dealing with another person's emotional fallout, especially if you're not used to dealing with it. We'd like to think that things won't get that bad, since we've added to this book all the failsafes

114

that we use to prevent such a drastic result in our own practice together, but never say never.

Pushing Limits

This brings us to the idea of limits, and just how far they can be "safely" pushed. Both magicians and kinky people may disagree with others of their ilk on how far is too far in their respective practices. More advanced forms of both are designed to really stretch the limits of the human psyche (and, depending on the situation, body).

We've been criticized for our uses of kink magic before, including being told that what we do is "too dangerous" and "should be left to professionals." Much of this is because when we work kink magic, it's very heavily psychological and is specifically designed to shatter the tunnel vision of one or more (willing) participants through an intense ritual. Understandably, this concept scares some people. We're sure that at least some of you reading this text will have a horror story or three about somebody who really fucked hirself up in either kink or magic (or both). Trust us — we have our stories, too.

However, we are responsible adults, and we hope you are, too! There are people out there who would love to see both kink and magic banned because they're supposedly "too dangerous" and "people might get hurt." These folks may mean well, but they ignore the fact that we are, in fact, responsible adults quite capable of making our own decisions about our bodies, minds and spirits. It is our opinion that the freedom of people to choose (at least in America) is already restricted enough; the government gets to decide what we should or shouldn't put in our bodies, the media and educational systems decide what we feed our minds, and some of the religions try to dictate what we should or should not nourish our spirits with. All of this is apparently for our own good, or so we're told.

Imagine having kink or magic banned, however, just because somebody decided that it was too dangerous for everyone involved, directly or indirectly. The occasional child custody cases that crop up when a person's less common sexual or religious practices are revealed would become more commonplace, and people might very well end up in prison just for what they desired or believed.

Now, we aren't trying to scare you into thinking that Orwell's *1984* is imminent. Our point is that we ask that you respect our

115

boundaries, as well as your own. If you find that something in here is too extreme for you, nobody's forcing you to go through with it.

We do intense work together. Both of us have used magic for years to consciously change ourselves. We've broken bad habits, rerouted unhealthy behavior patterns, and exorcised deeply-hidden demons in our psyches using kink and other forms of magic. We've done rape scenes to purge the effects of sexual assault, and "forced" each other to act out some of our deepest fears and insecurities.

However, we have gone through these things **only when we were ready to do so!** There is a fine line between teaching and torture. This is why we employ the safe word/action and communicate with each other on a frequent basis, both in and out of scenes, about things we'd like to work on, or are already changing on our own. **Neither one of us has ever pushed the other past the point where s/he felt ready to explore**.

Any tool can be used for constructive or destructive purposes. Humans have long misused pain and punishment to further their own bad conditioning by turning them on other humans for purposes of destruction. Rather than being used to rehabilitate people and teach them the effects of their destructive actions, punishment and pain have been used in the abuse of power with rehabilitation as an excuse. Our purpose here is to explore the constructive rather than destructive uses.

For example, let's look at the overlying dogma of the Catholic Church. For centuries, this religious body has threatened bad or "sinful" behavior with hellfire and damnation in the afterlife, and often with retribution in this life. The Inquisition was a primary example; those caught in its web were often no more than political prisoners who had done no true wrong, and they were subjected to horrific tortures in order to expiate their sins (and capture other sinners). This was often justified by the excuse that the flames of Hell would be much worse than the burning at the stake of this life.

Probably very few Inquisitors truly believed they were helping to purify their fellow human beings. We doubt there was a shortage of extreme sadists among that lot; given the frequency with which female (and occasionally male) prisoners were raped as a means of torture, the Inquisitors were not immune to the temptations of the flesh no matter how vile a manifestation thereof.

This attitude continues today. Children and adults alike cruelly taunt their peers, claiming to teach them a lesson about being socially abnormal in some way. It's obvious that the tormentors get a lot more pleasure than is warranted out of this, and very little rehabilitation occurs on the part of the target. The inhumane treatment of prisoners, too, is testament to our perception of punishment as being worthy only of "bad people" who are "beneath" their captors.

Yet, in true rehabilitation, the root cause is not to further destroy someone who is obviously already broken, but to raise them up to the level of their healthier peers. When punishment is applied in order to truly help the sufferer—whom we'll refer to henceforth as the initiate—the goal is not to break hir and leave hir broken so that s/he is no longer functional enough to cause further problems, but instead to break hir and reset hir in a healthier manner by hir will.

That is our basic philosophy in kink magic. When we take on the role of the torturer, the rapist, the predator, it is a device to trigger the suspension of disbelief that is so crucial to success in both scenes and rituals. No, it's not 100% safe, but what really is? This is a good example why we tend to like the RACK approach to kink magic. It's also why we have emphasized the importance of communication, knowing your limits and those of your partner(s), and knowing just who it is you're involved with and what everyone is doing. We can't make your decisions for you, but we can explain what has worked for us.

As we mentioned earlier, if you don't have any experience in purposely changing your psychology, pick up a couple of books by authors we recommended in Chapter 3. Authors such as Wilson and Lilly offer excellent resources to introduce you to the idea of conscious evolution.

Health and Preparation

So now that we've given you all the dire warnings, here are some ideas (along with all that communication) to help avoid emergencies.

Sex, in and of itself, can be a fairly strenuous activity, and when you add kink into the mix, a person's physical, emotional, psychological, and sometimes spiritual limits can be tested to the extreme. Kink magic can be a good workout, and warming up reduces the chances of both pulled muscles and psychological or energetic fuck-ups. We urge our readers to engage in a daily regimen of exercises and meditations unrelated to kink magic. While stretching may not look particularly sexy, tearing muscle tissue is even less so.

Physical exercise will help you tone your body and keep it in good shape. A conditioned body is less susceptible to pulled muscles and other structural strain. Additionally, the better shape you're in, the more energy you'll have, and the longer you can make your kink magic last. While we aren't medical experts or personal trainers, from our own experiences we've found that stretching muscles on a regular basis, and routine light cardiovascular exercise such as walking and aerobics, can go a long way in making a body feel better. Other common sense suggestions regarding health, including getting a good amount of sleep and eating a proper diet, will also further your efforts.

Just as your physical body needs exercise, so does your mind need mental exercise. Meditation disciplines and focuses your mind, and helps you to become more comfortable with ASCs. In addition, such exercises will also get you connected to your energetic body, which will prove useful when you bring energy work into play within kink magic. We suggest starting with *Relaxing into Your Being: Breathing, Chi, & Dissolving the Ego* by B. K. Frantzis if you've never meditated before, or would like a daily regimen to help maintain your current condition.

You can also try the following exercise: Sit comfortably in a chair with your hands on your lap and your feet flat on the floor. Take a deep breath in through your nose. The breath should be deep enough so that you push your belly out when you breathe in and pull it in when you breathe out. At the same time put the tip of your tongue on the roof of your mouth (in Taoist meditation, doing this completes the circuit of energy in your body). Now we want you to focus on your breathing. Don't think about anything else. Just keep inhaling and exhaling, feel and follow the motion of the breath. At first, as you do this exercise, you'll probably find yourself getting bored or thinking about random subjects. Do your best to keep your mind focused on the breathing. Eventually you'll find you get to a point where your awareness stays focused on the breathing. At that point, you will have experienced an ASC.

That experience may not seem particularly impressive at first, but if you continue doing the exercise daily, you'll likely find over time that you will be experiencing states of mind that are more dramatic. We also want to emphasize that the act of breathing is very important in achieving an ASC. This will become more evident later on in the book.

Meditation also aids greatly with relaxation. Being able to relax physically, emotionally, mentally, and spiritually will free up energy which can be put to excellent use. It is when you are most relaxed that you are simultaneously most receptive and most capable of directing magic. Relaxation is also essential for training the physical muscles of the body, so that exercise and other forms of wear don't damage them. Tense muscles lead to strain, pain, and stress, while relaxed muscles let all of the strain go. Additionally, relaxed muscles indicate that the natural energy of the body is flowing as opposed to being blocked. If you're afraid or have repressed emotions, that tension will show up in your muscles and create blockages that can interfere with your physical and emotional health.

Finally, on a more mundane level, there are a few things to keep with your first aid kit. If your kit doesn't have a pair of bandage scissors (the kind with nice blunt ends so you don't stab the flesh that you're releasing) you should invest in one in case the rope or other bonds won't come loose. Keep them sharp, too, especially if you use leather often. As we mentioned earlier, make sure there's a phone nearby; you can turn the ringer off, but in the case of a non-cellular phone don't unplug it! The last thing you need is for the top to have a heart attack and the bottom only able to reach the phone and not the plug. A list of emergency numbers is a good idea, too. Any medications that the participants might need should be close by as well, along with some protein-heavy food (beware of allergies) and water.

During the Scene

We've already touched on some of the issues to talk to your partner(s) about during the scene itself. A good rule of thumb[20] is for the top to routinely check on the possible causes of disasters every five to ten minutes or so. S/he doesn't actually have to say anything to the bottom unless there are signs of distress (bound extremities turning red, nails turning blue, consciousness fading, etc.). It's not too difficult to get into the habit of glancing at bondage implements periodically to make sure circulation is still good, or to make the bottom say something to be sure s/he's still coherent periodically without disrupting the scene or top space.

---

[20] Somewhat related to the topic at hand, the phrase "rule of thumb" didn't actually originate from an old English law stating that a man could beat his wife with any stick narrower than his thumb (the law doesn't exist). It springs instead from woodworkers who knew their trade well enough that they could literally measure with their thumbs. (Hiscock et al, 1993)

Granted, experienced tops will probably be used to keeping an eye on the bottom. However, it should never be taken for granted that everything's okay just because there's nothing overtly wrong. Additionally, familiarity can breed complacency even in experienced partners. And while the bottom might not be paying as much attention because s/he's zooming off into subspace, if s/he does notice something awry s/he needs to use the safe word/gesture as soon as s/he can, if possible.

It goes without saying that if any party uses the safe word/gesture, the scene needs to come to an immediate stop. This goes for scenes with more than two participants, too; even if the afflicted party leaves the room, the scene should not go on. First priority for everyone should be making sure that the reason the safe word/gesture was used is addressed immediately.

The same goes for any sort of physical medical emergency — cuts that were deeper than intended and won't stop bleeding, asthma attacks, light headedness, etc. Again, calling in an ambulance or rushing to the emergency room might be embarrassing, but having the EMTs laughing about you later on is an improvement over dealing with someone bleeding to death or passing out (and not waking up) in the dungeon.

If the issue can be resolved quickly ("Excuse me, but my pubic hair is stuck in the zipper on my leather undies — can you reach it for me?"), most people should have no trouble getting back into the scene. It may be incredibly annoying in the event that something irrevocably disrupts the scene, but we much prefer that possibility to the option of ignoring a potential problem.

Aftercare

Even in a scene that goes flawlessly with no harm done, it's still important to do aftercare. Along with the questions we listed above with regard to communication, it's a good idea to check everyone over at the conclusion of the scene. Inspect any bound or otherwise "tortured" body parts for actual damage, numbness, persistent pain beyond the usual, etc. Get some food and water into all participants to help ground them and assure proper hydration. Find a comfy place to sit (and maybe even cuddle) and talk about the scene, especially if anyone's feeling headspacey or upset. If things go wrong, refer to the section above on what to do.

Different people may have different requirements for aftercare. Some may want to snuggle, have small talk, and maybe even go to sleep in that safe, warm place. Others may want to have alone time, or go out somewhere to clear their heads from the ASC of the scene. Do whatever works; just make sure that all the participants check in to make sure everybody's okay. If a problem crops up later, make sure that whoever mentions it knows s/he can speak freely, no matter how seemingly insignificant the issue might be. It can sometimes take time for a problem to reveal itself, and what seems like a small thing may just be the tip of the iceberg.

You might also consider doing a banishing after the scene is done, even if it wasn't magical in nature. This helps to clear out residual energies from the play area, and also completes the grounding process. Doing the LBRP followed by a snack and some water tends to be a good practice, as it addresses the mental, emotional, spiritual, energetic and physical levels of the self. It shouldn't be a substitute for communication, just as magic shouldn't be a substitute for mundane efforts. Magic is used to augment mundane actions if used properly, and in this case it can contribute to a sense of security and groundedness.

You can't completely prevent mistakes, accidents, and "oh, fucks" from happening. However, what we've discussed are things that we've found will go a long way in keeping kink magic fun, effective, and out of the emergency room.

Chapter Eight: The Scene as Sacred Ritual Space

The word "ritual" has specific contexts and meanings, and doesn't always accurately describe the magical workings that a person may do. Before we provide our own definition of ritual, we want to examine some other perspectives on it:

--"Ritual has two uses (among many) that are important to how we get into states of ecstasy, how we travel safely, and how we get back out again. For our purposes, ritual can be like a container that defines the mental space we are operating in, and that protects that space, keeping it, and us, safe and inviolate" (Easton & Hardy 2004, p. 89). This definition argues that ritual provides a safe space in which different states of consciousness can be explored. It's certainly true that ritual can do this, but this definition is rather limited, at least as it applies to ritual and kink. Ritual does define a mental space, but it also defines other spaces.

--Ritual is also about sacred space. Eliade discusses how the creation of sacred space is equivalent to the creation of a world, "Revelation of a sacred space makes it possible to obtain a fixed point and hence acquire orientation in the chaos of homogeneity, to 'found the world' and to live in a real sense. The profane experience, on the contrary, maintains the homogeneity and hence the relativity of space" (1957, p.23). Sacred space is essential to the dynamic of ritual, and this also applies to kink. After all, in creating a scene, aren't we creating a liminal sacred space, a world all of its own outside the profane world?

--"Ritual is then described as particularly *thoughtless* action - routinized, habitual, obsessive, or mimetic and therefore the purely formal, secondary, and mere physical expression of logically prior ideas" (Bell 1992, p. 19). This particular definition of ritual would mechanize it. Obviously, ritual is not a thoughtless activity. If anything, ritual demands planning and a good sense of awareness and spontaneity. Ritual involves action, but also thought, albeit thought in an ASC. But Bell also points out that rituals involve practices, e.g. cultural activities, and that through these practices cultures are renegotiated (Bell 1992). This is important: we do ritual to renegotiate the boundaries in our lives and identities in order to find balance in our internal and external realities.

--Interestingly enough, Bell contradicts her idea of the thoughtless ritual in a later definition: "In ritual, it is probably safe to say that no act is purely manipulative or purely disinterested. Ritual acts of offering, exchange and communion appear to invoke very complex relations of mutual interdependence between the human and the divine. In addition, these activities are likely to be important not simply to human-divine relations but also to a number of social and cultural processes by which the community organizes and understands itself" (Bell 1997). Ritual is a way of connecting with the divine, the past, the environment, the community, and the sense of self. Placement of all these factors in ritual really can't be ignored because they all affect the creation of ritual and the purposes it is used for.

Ritual is a lot of things, and can even have multiple definitions for the same person. We haven't covered the full range of what ritual could be, but that's not the purpose of this book. The important thing to recognize is that ritual has a variety of different meanings, but how a ritual is defined can affect some of the magical workings you do.

However, formal ritual, such as that designed to honor the divine or to connect with community, isn't the limit of what magic, in general, can be. For example, when a person fires a sigil to find a job, it isn't a prerequisite that s/he be engaged in a ritual. Some people might argue that the choice to fire a sigil was a ritual in itself, but then the question is whether *everything* a person does is a ritual. We think it depends on the context and the perspective of the individual. For instance, brushing your teeth isn't usually perceived as a ritual, but it could be with a different angle of perception – repetition is ritual. Ritual, in the magical/religious sense, is based off the meanings people read into activities they consider to be a part of the ritual space they inhabit when taking part in ritual. Brushing teeth isn't considered a ritual because it isn't perceived as a liminal activity, i.e. an activity that occurs in sacred space, that place which falls between conventional reality and the unknown.

Some would argue that any act of magic is a ritual, even wanking to the point of orgasm over a paper sigil. However, in our understanding of the term, ritual conveys a certain sense of preparation and formality. The individual interpretations and

124

expressions may vary, but there is a certain level of Importance-with-a-big-I that sets rituals apart from, say, spells or simple sigil casting. Rituals often have at least some formulaic elements that help to set the stage and trigger the ASC in the minds of all participants.

Again, for some people this can and will be different, but context shapes what ritual can be for each person, and it's up to each person to decide what ritual means to hir. For this book in particular, we define ritual as the establishment of the scene in the kink magic context.

Our Definition of Ritual: The Scene as Ritual Space

When we think of a scene, we think of it as a ritual. It's a liminal space, a place that doesn't exist in an ESC or linear time/space. The perception of time slows down so that while an hour passes, to the participants it might feel like it's been three hours. This disconnection from linear time is a part of ritual and is a way of knowing that the ritual space, or sacred space, has been established.

The scene is also liminal in that the physical space it occurs in is usually a private or personal space. This is also true for rituals. People who attend a specific ritual are typically invited, and are part of the cultural community in which the ritual takes place. In the case of the BDSM/kink community, we meet at dungeons, bedrooms in our homes, private residences, or other places away from public. Thus, the physical space of a scene is liminal because only certain people can enter that space, and the activities that occur there stay there.

This extends to mental space as well. Through a combination of play and props, sensations and stimulation, a person is brought to an ASC. That altered state can be used to work changes in a person's psyche, or to change external circumstances via practical magic. We use this state of consciousness to effect change because it focuses a person, making them more aware of possibilities than they would be in an ESC. Additionally, the accompanying suspension of disbelief removes mental blockages that can prevent us from accepting "irrational" ideas (such as the crazy idea that magic actually works!).

On a spiritual level, we can use the ASC to connect with the gods, spirits, and hidden aspects of ourselves that we might otherwise avoid or not know how to access. The scene becomes a spiritual space when we choose to use it for magical purposes, whether those purposes include a guided pathworking, an initiation, or a practical magical working. People practicing BDSM alone have obtained spiritually moving experiences, as well, with no magic involved.

Finally, the scene is sacred space because it's a world we create. That created world has its own reality, and for the duration of our play, it is the only one we exist in. It establishes boundaries against the ESC and, through the props and costumes, a mythology of its own. We see this in standard BDSM scenes, even if the participants don't consciously recognize it. The choice of a specific role as a top or a bottom carries with it a variety of meanings that help to establish the power dynamic; the world is created by the needs and desires of all parties to be satiated through that dynamic.

Ritual, with or without kink, is motivated by need and desire for sacred space and all it entails. Whether that desire is to celebrate the gods or to create deep internal change, it creates the world of the ritual and establishes a connection within, without, or both. It's important to recognize these different aspects of ritual in the scene, because through such recognition we can intentionally use the scene to accomplish a desired end.

So Is a Scene Really a Ritual?

A scene *can* be a magically-focused ritual, but it doesn't have to be. Some people in the kink community will have no interest in working sex magic into BDSM. So is their scene a ritual? It depends partially on how they perceive their actions, but also depends on the intent going into it. People who are just playing with each other for fun aren't likely to think of their scene as a ritual. However, people who go into a scene with the intent of invoking a god or casting a spell or sigil as part of the scene will likely consider it to be a ritual, at least on some level.

We do want to note that a scene, whether it's intended as a ritual or not, will always share certain characteristics with what defines a ritual. The creation of a liminal space, the focus on a desired goal, and the ASC are similarities that scenes share with rituals. But what makes a scene into a ritual is the choice and intent of everyone involved.

There are no set criteria for determining if a scene is a ritual beyond the intent of all parties going into the scene. However, everyone involved must be aware that a ritual will be performed.

Working sex magic with someone who doesn't know what's going on is generally considered unethical, and in our opinion, it's dangerous to all parties. Its better that each person has the option of choosing not to participate than to secretly do a ritual with someone who normally wouldn't consent to it. The psychological and energetic harm that can result, if the person realizes what is occurring, will not be a pretty sight. Even if s/he doesn't consciously realize what happened, there can be negative fallout that s/he may not be able to explain, but which affects hir nonetheless.

So why do people use ritual in kink? Easton and Liszt offer one answer:

> Ritual S/M is edge play directed to the purpose of attaining altered states of consciousness, of traveling beyond our habitual perceptual screens to another way of being in which everything becomes special, extraordinary, brilliant. Goals for such a scene might be a quest for guidance, or a vision, the pursuit of personal truth and understanding, or the experience of spiritual communion for its own sake. (1995, p. 148)

These are certainly good reasons for doing ritual, though not the only reasons. Other reasons can include practical purposes, such as manifesting a certain desire into physical reality, or healing purposes, such as allowing a person to confront a part of hir past, thereby healing previous personal damage.

Sceners also use rituals for communication, and for creating stronger bonds among the participants. Good rituals involve honest communication with yourself, your partner(s), and any other beings worked with. Only when we can freely open ourselves and give willingly to the ritual, can we in turn receive from the ritual. A closed heart and mind will shut down a ritual faster than anything else.

Another reason for the crossover between kink and magical ritual is the ease with which you can attain an ASC through kink. Sub space and top space fall under the ASC heading; your view of reality is quite different during a scene, regardless of whether you're the bottom or the top. The sensory overload of heavy whipping or other hyperstimulation can send the recipient flying off (mentally) into other realms, provided it's done with an eye toward achieving a specific state. But a ritual just isn't a ritual without the ASC, regardless of what trappings you use.

The Importance of ASCs

As we mentioned earlier, an altered state of consciousness varies from the general "autopilot" mundane consciousness that we generally have. ASCs can range from having an out of body experience, to being so connected to something or someone other than yourself that you temporarily "become" it, to simply feeling incredibly relaxed and in a state of half sleep. An ASC can also be a transcendent state that provides a lot of energy, which can be used for any purpose the person chooses (Easton & Hardy 2004). This allows us access to what are often termed "supernatural" phenomena, including the practice of magic. Without an ASC, even a mild one, a ritual is only a person pantomiming certain movements; the ASC turns it from mere pretending into actual manifestations of change.

Bringing someone to an ASC through kink isn't just a matter of flogging them bloody:

> The kind of pain that works best as a tool of altered states...should be able to be sustained at the same level for a long period of time, or be adjustable as needed. It should not cause too much in the way of physical damage, because that might make you pass out and miss the entire experience. It's carefully controlled, carefully orchestrated pain, not random flailing, and the best way to work with it is to do it slowly and with attention to the reaction of one's body. (Kaldera 2006, p. 27)

Kaldera's example shows that entering an ASC using kink involves some sophistication and awareness of impact. An ASC must be delicately cultivated, even if the methods themselves are anything but gentle, as the state can easily by shattered by the wrong action. This is why it's a bad idea to bring up this week's grocery list in the middle of a psychologically heavy scene (unless, of course, the bottom is being chastised for forgetting to run errands). In most cases, killing the mood also kills the ASC.

The pain and other stimuli should be used with an awareness of a person's limits, and with an eye toward moving past those limits *carefully*, if at all. Nothing will snap a person out of an ASC quicker than having their limits rudely (and non-consensually) crossed. For example, Lupa *hates* anything cold. Introducing ice to her skin in any scene would not only wake her out of her ASC, but would put a swift end to that play session! Granted, some people hit deeper ASCs when subjected to things they normally hate. However, it shouldn't be assumed that it's okay to push certain buttons -- that sort of edgeplay needs to be reserved for those who have been playing together for a long time and who understand both how far their partner(s) can be pushed, and what to do if it goes too far.

Using psychological triggers can also create an ASC, if particularly sensitive issues are used. For example, in one ritual we'll elaborate on later, Taylor deliberately invoked and embodied the qualities of a psychologically-abusive ex-boyfriend of Lupa's. This caused her to recall the feelings she'd had during that relationship, and allowed her to use her subsequent growth to heal the remaining scars. Instead of cowering in fear as she once would have, she took control and banished the ill effects of that relationship. This is a common method we use with each other, with great success, though it's something we usually plan in advance.

ASCs aren't limited to the bottom, though, as one might assume. It can be incredibly difficult for the top to be a cruel bitch or bastard, especially if that's a part of hirself s/he is not particularly comfortable with. Both of us have, on occasion, needed aftercare after topping each other in particularly vicious scenes ("Oh, my gods, what have I done to my poor mate?!"). However, at such times, we access parts of ourselves that we don't normally use in an everyday context.

Proper breathing is essential to ASCs. Breath circulates the natural energy of the body, while also stimulating physiological changes -- both of which can lead to ASCs. Fast in-and-out breathing is known as bellows, continuous, or pranic breathing, and is one way to enter an ASC. Bellows breathing is different from hyperventilating, because it's controlled. It's used to build-up a person's internal energetic cycle and can synchronize one person's energetic cycle with another's. It's a circular breathing. You inhale and then exhale without taking a pause between the exhale and inhale.

The water meditation breathing techniques written about by B. K. Frantzis have been particularly helpful for Taylor. This technique combines slower, deeper breaths with energy work to break down energetic blockages or tension points that repress emotions. As these blockages are dissolved, the emotions are expressed and processed. This is an intensive process involving facing one's inner demons, but as the energy dissolves and the emotions are expressed, the person gradually finds balance (Frantzis 2001). We've used this technique for our synchronized breathing work. It does an excellent job of relaxing the muscles and stimulating the energy of the body, and can be very helpful when working through traumatic issues.

Regardless of what style of breath training you use, the key is to use the diaphragm to breathe, which helps to exercise the full capacity of the lungs, as opposed to just the upper chest. When you're focusing on the act of breathing, the sensations help to teach the proper discipline necessary for quieting the mind enough to work magic successfully. Additionally, breath training teaches you to be aware of the internal rhythms of the body, which is key to working with your internal energy.

Both/all participants may reach mild ASCs prior to ritual by synchronizing their breathing. Take a few minutes to face each other, sitting or standing, and breathe together. This may also be used during the scene itself; the top may order the bottom to pay attention to how the top breathes as a way of bringing the bottom's focus back to the scene if s/he's getting too spacey, or if extra attention needs to be paid to the working. Alternately, rhythmically flogging a person can set up a breathing pace that puts participants into an ASC. The sensation and sound of flogging can be a breathing metronome, especially if the top is skilled at keeping a rhythm for an extended period. Those who integrate music into their scenes will find this rhythm an acceptable substitute.

Breathing in synchronization is important not just in a physiological sense, but on an energetic level as well. It connects the energy of the participants through the parallel physical functions affecting the energetic body. When people are connected on one level (such as the energetic), it carries over into others (physical, psychological, etc). This is why people may refer to a scene as "having good energy." We experience reality through multiple types of perception, not just our physical senses.

On the other hand, hyperventilation can occur, especially if a person is deeply shocked while in subspace. At that point, it's important for the top to take control of the situation and get the bottom's breathing back under control. When either of us hyperventilates, the other one helps hir control hir breathing by gently grabbing hir hair and telling hir to slow hir breathing. We both take deep, slow breaths until we are both calm and ready to either renew the scene or stop for the night.

Regardless of *how* you shift your consciousness, the ability to shift is crucial to successful rituals. Rituals shake your foundation in ways that you'd never encounter otherwise. This necessitates the ability to view the world, at least temporarily, from the vantage point of an ASC. Without it, no changes occur on any level, and you may as well be reading lines from an uninspired script to an audience of blowup dolls, accompanied by the sound of water dripping from a leaky faucet.

Taking Advantage of That Long, Strange Trip

Once you've reached an ASC, it's time to project your intent and desire into reality. It's important that you have the goal and target(s) clearly in mind, and that you stay focused on them. The goal is the desire itself, and its manifestation. The target is the process or mechanism that will allow that manifestation to occur. For instance, if your goal is to find a new job, your targets are your resume, and the potential employers you must convince to hire you. The ASC is where the process begins, as it aligns your internal awareness with the external reality, allowing you to take advantage of possibilities that come your way.

Let's run with the job analogy for a bit. Suppose the job seeker has been having trouble with hir confidence, making it hard to really get out and make things happen. The analogous resume is partially completed but in need of updating, and the email addresses of headhunters are just sitting in the address book, rather than being used to communicate with job agencies. At the heart of this is the job seeker, who is insecure and deeply terrified of a new job. S/he fears miserably failing her job interviews. Instead of applying for jobs s/he's qualified for, s/he's telling hirself, "It won't work, so why try at all?"

If s/he happens to be a bottom, hir top could get hir into a deep ASC by playing on those fears. The top might force hir to confess all the terrors and insecurities; or s/he might indulge in a little roleplay and get creative with the interview process. Either way, the point is to bring all the reasons s/he's not job hunting to the surface. Once that's accomplished, the top might force the bottom to see how ridiculous hir reasons are. The top could end that section of the ritual with the bottom explaining why s/he's a good choice for the job, thereby working to banish the fear. Alternately, soft topping might include the top performing a healing ritual to gently banish the negative thoughts and replace them with assertive ones. S/he could even require the bottom to act out a mock job interview.

There are possibilities for the job seeker to act as a top as well. In this case, the bottom would represent the top's fears, perhaps by repeating the top's insecure statements during the ritual. The top might then take control of the situation through the bottom. In a hard topping situation, s/he might flog the bottom to exorcise those fears (which may actually be easier for some, as it temporarily distances the top from the emotions so that they don't control hir). Or, during soft topping, s/he might explain to the bottom why s/he's hurting hirself with these painful thoughts—and in the process, learning why they are harmful to hir attempts to find a job.

The above situations are just examples of ASCs being used to bring desire into reality. Many people have a difficult time dealing with problems in ESC, such as our theoretical job seeker who sabotages hirself on a daily basis. But once s/he's in that ASC, s/he's able to access healthier behavior patterns. The process of job hunting, which was stunted by fear in our above example, is changed for the better within the more fluid, liminal sacred space. It's not that these changes couldn't be wrought in ESC—but the ASC makes it easier and more effective.

Regardless of our backgrounds, our tastes, and our trances, there is a need for ritual. We use it celebrate our lives, resolve our conflicts, and set our notions of reality right. When a society has no ritual, it misses out on the connection of life. This is why Western culture has become so stagnant. We have no central mythos, no cultural heroes, and we often hide behind technological advances that only sever us from the rest of reality. Yet, we can escape for only so long. Finding ritual is finding connection and communication with ourselves and other people, and that's why we think ritual fits well with kink -- because whether you're in a dungeon, at a play party, or in a bedroom, you are sharing a level of intimacy rarely experienced elsewhere.

Chapter Nine: Practical Magic

Practical magic is magic utilized for mundane, everyday purposes. This is what is known in some circles as "low" magic, concerned primarily with creating change on an everyday basis (as opposed to "high" magic, which is concerned with transcendence). Most spells and sigils, as well as the bulk of pre-crafted rituals found at the neopagan/witchcraft end of the magical spectrum, are in this category. We don't believe practical magic is inherently inferior (or superior) to metamorphic magic—just different in its focus and purpose.

Curiously enough, the available literature on kink magic doesn't extensively cover practical magic. Most esoteric approaches to BDSM tend toward spirituality; magical uses focus primarily on metamorphic magic. We don't think that kink magic should be limited to inner transformation, particularly when some of the material is so well suited to practical application.

Take fetishes, for example. Fetishes, by their nature, require a great deal of focus, even to the point of obsession, and it's a relatively simple task to turn that focus to a magical purpose. One of our examples in this chapter involves applying a sigil to the object of one's desire, and using fetishistic attention to add energy to that focus. Everybody has plenty of fun, but you're also accomplishing something more mundane.

Here are some examples of practical ways we've used kink magic. Obviously, you're not limited to these; as with the rest of this book, this chapter is meant to get your mental cogs grinding away on ideas and applications of your own.

Evocation and Invocation

The stereotypical being called in sex magic evocation is an incubus or succubus. These entities feed on energy generated by the act of sex (U.D. 2001). They are astral lovers for magicians, and in exchange for sexual energy, one can have them accomplish specific tasks. However, magicians have also taken other entities, including deities, as spiritual sex partners over the centuries. There's a risk of obsession in working with entities in this manner, mainly because you are sharing such intimate energy with them. It's dangerous particularly for those with unsatisfactory sex lives, as the entity can replace the desire for an actual human partner (to include the healthy, nonsexual social interaction with a human partner)[21].

You can bypass this obsession: instead of having direct sexual interaction with the entity, have it draw on the ambient energy generated by a scene. (Make sure everyone involved knows beforehand what's going on.) Use the energy of the pain and pleasure to express the task you want the entity to accomplish. The bottom should imprint every sensation s/he feels with that task, and the same goes for the top's focus while inflicting those sensations. The energy generated by the physical activity and attention to the stimulation is fed to the entity, programming it to do the task. You might visualize the entity materializing in the energy rising from the bodies of the participants, or send the energy into a vessel the entity may use as a temporary physical anchor for the duration of the ritual. Remember to use the ambient energy to call up the entities, and not your own energy. If you use your own energy, the entities will draw on that instead of the ambient energy, which can drain you as it feeds.

You're not limited to incubi and succubae, of course; evocation may involve Goetic demons, deities, spirits, and/or any other type of entity a person can think of. There are numerous purposes for evocation, too. In addition to our example of summoning a being to complete a particular task, you might instead evoke an entity associated with sex and/or pain (there are numerous deities who fit the bill one or both ways) to add their energy to a kink magic ritual. You could evoke entities associated with protection to guard the ritual area during the scene, especially if you are going to be addressing vulnerable issues. You could call upon healing entities at the close of a ritual, to help bring everyone back into a calm, secure state of mind.

If you can't find an entity for your purpose, there's always the option of creating one. We designed a magical species on the astral plane called a sigilonodon. This is a lizard-like creature that captures energy with webbed membranes stretched down the sides of its body between its fore- and back legs. It collects and stores energy within itself until called upon for magical use. Each

---

[21] There are healthy cases of people having spiritual/magical relationships with nonphysical entities. One of the (relatively) better-known examples is the lwa marriage in Vodou. It's not uncommon for members of that religion to marry one or more lwa, whether or not the human already has a physical significant other (Filan 2007).

sigilonodon has a large scale between its shoulder blades; on it, we inscribe a sigil representing what we want to accomplish.[22] We created the first sigilonodon with kink magic because sex represents the creative force, and being who we are, we wanted to incorporate aspects of kink into the working.

We created the necessary ASC through overstimulation, using, among other things, a mind machine. First, Taylor bound Lupa's arms and legs so her movement was restricted, spreading her legs enough for cunnilingus. Then he put the goggles and headphones of the mind machine on her. Taylor stimulated Lupa sexually, instructing her to focus her mind and energy on the creation and evocation of the magical species.

Taylor focused on the sexual act, generating energy for the birth of the sigilonodon. We found that the binding of Lupa's limbs, along with the physical input provided by the oral sex and the mind machine, resulted in an excellent method for creating and evoking an entity. The overstimulation via the mind machine gave Lupa enough noise and light to achieve gnosis and open her mind to the process of creating the entity. The sexual energy from the cunnilingus and the resulting orgasm collected in her solar plexus chakra, which we then used to create the first sigilonodon.

We also approach evocation as a way of manifesting possibility into reality. It might seem that we are doing an enchantment, but we think evoking a possibility is more accurate. In evocation, we are calling into external reality a possibility, with potential unknown variables. Conversely, enchantment involves working with known and present variables that we manipulate to maximize their effectiveness.

We can evoke events with the same techniques we use to evoke entities, including the ambient energy method. In this case, you program the energy raised through ritual activity to evoke the possibility, allowing it to manifest into your life. Evoking possibilities and events requires you to rely heavily on your intuition. As an example, Taylor wanted to meet local pagans in Kent, Ohio when he first moved there. He evoked the possibility of making contacts within the community. After the ritual was complete, whenever his intuition prompted him to do something and he acted upon it, he would meet another pagan in the area.

---

[22] Lupa extensively covers how to create and work with a magical species in her book *Fang and Fur, Blood and Bone: A Primal Guide to Animal Magic*.

A kinkier version of this type of evocation has the bottom focus all of hir energy and attention on the possibility to be evoked. S/he visualizes the possibility during the scene, using the pain and pleasure to feed the desired outcome. When it is fully visualized, the bottom will mentally pull that possibility into reality. When we do this, we visualize the possibility as a bubble, which we then mentally manifest into our reality. When the merging is complete, the bubble pops and reality changes so the possibility can manifest. Orgasm is particularly useful for merging the bubble into reality, as then the bottom's attention is most concentrated and yet at a non-linear nexus point where s/he can perceive the effect of the merging.

While, strictly speaking, evocation means calling forth an entity outside of the magician, evocation may even be paired with invocation, with one participant (generally the top) evoking the entity into the body of another participant (usually the bottom, though if there is a second top involved s/he may also be a vessel). The top may also invoke an entity hirself.

You may even use a scene as an offering to an entity that has successfully finished a task. The energy of the scene, as mentioned above, can be offered in honor of the entity. If knifeplay is involved, you may offer the blood, and if desired, leave a small scar as a reminder of the experience. Or, if all parties agree to it, the entity may even be invoked into a participant, so s/he may participate more directly in the offering process.

Regardless of who and what you evoke, make sure that you banish after the working is over. This is particularly true of entities such as incubi and succubae that may continue feeding on energy as long as there is available access.

Sigils

Sigils are forms of evocation, in a sense, as they evoke certain possibilities. Sigils interact with the subconscious mind on a symbolic level to create conditions through which the desired reality can manifest. We've taken some intriguing approaches to sigilization in kink magic.

Pain is an excellent source of energy to charge sigils with. A common practice is to tape a copy of the sigil to the wall or another place where the bottom can see it, and then get the scene underway. One time Lupa used a combination of pain and sensual pleasure to induce Taylor to charge a sigil, making him keep his eyes on it the entire time. As he reached his limits, she counted to ten, striking him as she counted. At the end of the count, Taylor released the sigil loaded with all the energy of the scene.

One approach we use is to put a sigil on a mirror, applying the fetish of narcissism. One of the most exciting sights for a narcissist is watching hirself being fucked by someone focused on hir pleasure.

Lupa Speaks:

Can I just say that I love mirrors? I'm vain, I admit it. I like seeing how I look, whether I'm dressed up or down, from different angles. I'll even sneak glances in storefront windows. And, of course, I love watching myself have sex. I've got a twenty-four-inch-diameter round mirror hanging over the head of our bed. I've gotten good mileage out of it, and it's been a popular toy among my lovers.

I've used mirrors to cast sigils before, though in a different capacity. One memorable ritual involved my drawing a sigil on a mirror and then trying to see my image through it. My narcissism, in a nonsexual context, got the best of me. I became so annoyed at having the sigil in the way of what I wanted to see that I lost my temper and clawed it into a blur of pink smudges.

One evening, Taylor made use of my narcissism to cast a sigil for a joint venture of ours. He had me design the sigil and draw it on the mirror over the bed. He then topped me rather roughly, drawing out a good bit of energy in the process and focusing it into the sigil. There was nothing unusual in this, but then he positioned me so I could watch us in the mirror. I focused on my reflection through the sigil, entranced by my own image and further stimulated by connecting the visual image with the touch-sensations I was experiencing. I then saw why Taylor had included the mirror sigil. I observed, through my libido-raging haze, that the energy we were building not only passed back and forth between us and our reflections, but charged the sigil with each pass. This noticeably enhanced the magic *and* our physical arousal. The physical and energetic dynamics fed each other, and the result was a thoroughly exhausted (but happy!) bottom and a successfully charged sigil.

Taylor Speaks:

I'm not really a narcissist. While I enjoy occasionally looking at myself and preening over my appearance, my attention is usually elsewhere, like on Lupa, who likes my attention focused on her. Even when I'm topping her, I focus on her pleasure, and when she tops me, it's for her pleasure and at her pace. Though we consider ourselves switches as opposed to strict D/s, this dynamic still informs our interactions.

Because she's narcissistic, I like using the mirror in our play. When I top her, I'll make her look at herself as I flog or punish her. I'll hold her hair just tightly enough to make her look at herself. When I bottom to her, I'll position myself so she can see herself in the mirror. I'll focus my eyes on her face and body, looking at her and sending my adoration into her. Seeing this in the mirror turns her on, because she knows I'm focused on her to the exclusion of everything else, including myself. This energy is directed to her and then to the sigil, charging it, while also building her sexual pleasure.

Any fetish can be utilized in this manner. Simply draw, paint or otherwise inscribe the sigil on the object desired, and use the attention to that item to charge the magic. You can utilize the energy in attention in non-fetishistic ways, as well; for example, the top may order the bottom to keep hir visual focus on the sigil throughout the scene, with dire consequences if hir attention wavers.

One of our other favorite materials for inscribing sigils is body paints. We use the body paints as a sensual approach to kink, and as highly useful forms of expression and appreciation for the other person. The body makes a wonderful canvas for painted sigils, which we can then use for a variety of magical operations. We paint sigils for invocations, providing a pathway for the entity to follow to establish contact with the targeted person.

The best time to apply sigils is before the scene starts, as this gives the paint time to dry, ensuring easier clean up and making the sigils themselves more durable. If including pain play in the scene, paint the symbols where they won't be hit, and avoid painting areas that will be bound. (An exception would be if you wanted to cast the sigil by flogging it off the bottom's skin. In this instance, consider that casting the sigil may take a while, and you'll need to clean the flogger—and the bottom—off later.). Both the top and the bottom may wear sigils, charging them with the energy of the scene.

We recommend the water soluble paint found at costume stores or, failing that, acrylics. Both are easy to wash off skin with soap and water, and dry quickly. If acrylic paint gets on clothes, carpets or sheets, it will be permanent. When you shower and wash the paints off, you are purifying yourself of evoked/invoked energies.

Another fun approach to sigils in kink magic is to make your partner try to assume a physical position that depicts the sigil. The harder it is to assume the position, the better, as the effort will force the person to focus that much more. The person must then hold this position for as long as possible. Hir efforts will charge the sigil, as will any punishments the top inflicts in the meantime. This could make for fun torture involving temperatures, tickling, and oral or manual stimulation!

Alternately, you could chant a word sigil as a mantra during a punishment -- instead of counting with numbers, the bottom could call out the mantra with each stroke. The top could instruct the bottom to personify the sigil, including painting it on the bottom's body, and using the mantra version in place of the bottom's actual name. Participants can call out the sigil at the moment of one participant's orgasm, while visualizing it to help direct energy toward the goal. The more focus placed on the sigil, the better.

Divination

We approach divination as more an act of shaping the future, rather than foreseeing the future. This resembles our definition of evocation. The very act of perceiving an event changes it, which is why it's better to focus on manifesting the most ideal outcome than to accept whatever your tarot cards (or other divinatory device) proclaim. For example, Lupa has habitually begun to turn tarot cards that predict misfortunate, afterward meditating on ways she can change that possibility; this helps to manifest the desired outcome rather than the unwanted one.

Sex magic is an effective method of divination. "The orgasm is often a strongly visionary experience, and it therefore makes sense to use sex magic to support this 'clairvoyance.' The post-orgasmic phase is especially conducive to visions" (U.D. 2001, p. 87). Taylor has experienced these visions, often finding himself in a place where he can observe and work with multiple possibilities for a specific event. At orgasm, Taylor relaxes into this ASC, allowing his mind to fill with possibilities. He equates it to being in a place of liquid and crystalline possibilities. He chooses the event that most suits his need and pulls it into reality (as mentioned in the evocation section). He feels like a nexus point in a web with the ability to go to any other point in the web, then become that point. By using this method, Taylor changes divination from an act of perception to one of enchantment. The movement from one point of reference to another allows Taylor to assume the new possibility in his life.

Sensory deprivation works well for divination because it forces the recipient to focus on hir thoughts, rather than on physical motion or other external distractions. Here's an example:

Taylor Speaks:

One evening, Lupa and I were discussing personal issues she had with her past, and how she deals with them. She was already in a meditative state, using me as a sounding board by sharing her feelings and answering my questions. Eventually, she started to offer excuses as her replies, instead of seeking constructive answers. I challenged her on these excuses, and when she continued to offer them, I took action. I slapped her across the face, pushing her out of meditation.

Using the shock from the slap, I told her that excuses weren't getting to the root of the problems, and that if she intended to work through the issues, she needed to do a divination that would allow her to interact with the issues on a deeper level. I put leather cuffs on her legs and arms, and covered her body with a blanket. I then left the room, turned off the light and closed the door, isolating her from me and from other distractions.

When I bound her arms to the bed, I made sure to use a clasp that would allow her to free herself if she so chose. This way she could enter her divinatory meditation and get answers she needed without interruption; however, I made it clear that doing so was her choice. I could have increased the sensory deprivation with a blindfold and other contrivances, but even without that, it worked well and helped her achieve a state of mind where she could divine the root causes of her issues and work out solutions to them.

Lupa Speaks:

I can be stubborn (something that frustrates and amuses my mate to no end), so when I wanted him with me during a meditation on some tough issues, and he tried changing the direction, I wasn't initially cooperative. He knows what buttons to push by now, and so was able to get me into a light sub space with the right tone of voice and a few slaps.

I haven't done much with sensory deprivation; I'm a bigger fan of overstimulation, through dance, sex magic and other activities. Still, this was a good experience for me, once my initial indignity wore off. I'm usually so active and busy that I don't always take the time needed to examine things internally as closely as I should.

While I was lying there in four-point restraints, covered in a blanket and restricted from doing anything but thinking, I went through a range of emotions. First, I was angry that he'd dare do such a thing to me (though I had agreed to it). Then, I became upset as the weight of the issues, and the fact that I had to deal with them alone, hit me full force. Finally, resignation set in, and I dug into what was bothering me. After a while, I reached a conclusion, finding constructive material for future meditations. At that point, I freed myself, knowing that I no longer needed the restraints to force me to think about my situation.

The second approach to divination is sensory overstimulation. With this approach, the senses are stimulated to the extreme in order to produce divinatory visions or connections. While the methods vary, the person performing the divination is forced to narrow hir focus to a particular point. The ASC from overstimulation may cause a more headspacey state of mind than deprivation, but if the recipient receives a question or other focus prior to the ritual, s/he can use it to keep from mentally floating off into the uncharted aethers. In these states, we sometimes use bondage gear, because although the gear restricts movement, it's another sensation that we can use to add to the overall stimulation.

Other sensations we can use vary from temperature to pressure, to pain, to sensual touching. For instance, we've used hot wax and ice to provide temperature differences. We've placed objects on the body (such as stones, blocks, feathers, pillows, etc) for gentle pressure (or lack thereof). We've inflicted varying degrees of pain with floggers, knives, paddles, pinwheels and other such toys. For sensual touching, we have used feathers, the tracing of a nail or fingertip on skin, and even a strip of fur. We'll usually mix and match these different sensations to provide a wide range of sensation, all of which is focused on pushing the person's sense of touch over the edge.

Another approach we've taken with this has sometimes involved restricting one sense while focusing on other senses, as sort of combination stimulation/deprivation. Sight is the sense that's easiest to restrict; simply tie a blindfold over the person's eyes. You can also restrict hearing by using earplugs or headphones to muffle noise. Touch can be constrained by bondage gear and a blanket; taste and smell are more difficult, though taste may be partially restricted with a gag. It's generally not a good idea to cover both the nose and the mouth (unless you like asphyxiation play, which we don't), for general safety reasons. We tend to favor incorporating smell and taste into this kind of working, because they aren't used as much (outside of eating). Feeding a person different flavors or bringing them different items to smell can titillate the senses and be a very novel experience. The recipient may notice that smell and taste are much more versatile than they previously realized.

When one sense is constrained, the other senses become sharper. The bottom might be nervous about what s/he is missing with regard to the restricted sense, but this can also heighten hir awareness. This is especially true with sight, which we often rely on almost to the exclusion of other senses. With the recipient deprived of sight, you can play with hir other senses in unexpected ways. For instance, paddle or flog hir with a rhythmic beat, and then vary the timing. This removes predictability and causes hir to feel uncertain, on top of the other sensations s/he is feeling, as s/he has no idea when the next blow will land.

One of our favorite tools for overstimulation is the mind machine. The audiostrobe technology bombards the sight and hearing senses of the recipient, causing a swift state of overstimulation. Below, we relate an example of how we used the mind machine with other sensations for some divinatory magic.

Taylor Speaks:

Lupa topped me for this session. I was doing visionary divinatory work with the Earth chakra as part of a long-term elemental ritual, in which I dedicate myself to a specific element for a year. In October 2006, I chose to work with the Earth element, as I felt ungrounded at the time. I wanted to do a divination to meet with the earth elemental spirits I'd be working with, to determine whether this element was the right choice for me. I'd noticed that my usually successful, conventional methods of meditation hadn't been very useful. I needed a different approach that would help me reach a deep enough ASC to get me where I needed to go.

Lupa had me lie on my belly with my arms underneath the pillow supporting my head. I'm not usually comfortable lying on my stomach, but the discomfort I felt made me aware of my body, something I correlated to the Earth element. She then had me put the goggles and headphones on and turn on the mind machine. As the sounds came on, the strobe lights activated, providing me with a kaleidoscope of shifting patterns and images. At the same time, she began to rub a pierce of fur on my body. At times, she'd switch to paddling me, but eventually settled on massaging me with some shea butter for my dry (and by then somewhat sore) skin. This was very cooling and relaxing.

The combination of sound, touch and sight helped put me into a deeply relaxed state. I was able to meditate on the astral gateway to the Earth Elemental plane and actually go meet the elemental spirits to get the information I needed for the best course of action.

Lupa Speaks:

This was something I'd wanted to play with for a while. The mind machine is a fun toy all around, but I wanted to see how it would mesh with overstimulation of the skin, something Taylor tends to react well to on its own.

I was quite pleased when he began to relax under the dual stimuli of the mind machine and the sensations I was introducing to his skin. I often alternate between pain and pleasure, partly to give his nerves some variety so they don't become too used to any one sensation, and partly to keep him (mentally) on his toes. I didn't want to disturb the magic he was working, so I just kept up the sensual play until he began to move around again.

One technique that I attempted was timing the skin stimulation in conjunction with the strobe in the goggles. I was kneeling to one side of him, and I could see the lights in the space between the goggles and his face. It's a lot tougher than it looks! It kept things challenging, especially since this was a low-key ritual for me, as I was mostly concerned with keeping Taylor off in happy-divination-land rather than directly interacting with him on a conscious level.

While people usually assume that the bottom will be the person subjected to deprivation or stimulation, the top may be the diviner, as well. This is why we referred to the "recipient" above. The top may have hir bottom(s) prepare hir for divination, acting as magical servants. The bottom(s) may even treat the top as a divine being, using worship to get hir into the mood for the magic and preparing hir for hir journey. The top retains control, even as s/he is restricted or punished; s/he may require more pain, or the closing off of another sense. On the other hand, some techniques, such as those involving psychological uncertainty due to deprivation, may be better suited to bottoms.

In kink magic, the deprivation approach and the overstimulation approach to divination work equally well. We like to use both approaches interchangeably, but some people might prefer one or the other, depending on the kink they prefer. Regardless, both approaches are useful for creating ASCs that allow the bottom to do effective divination.

Energy Work

Other than the sigil work described above, in the practical applications of kink magic, the top primarily uses energy work to steer and direct the energy of the bottom. It helps if the practitioner is aware of the different energetic systems of magic. In sex magic, we tend to favor three particular methods to energy work.

The first method is an aggressive approach where the top creates a cycle of energy, passing it back and forth between hir and the bottom. The purpose of the cycling is to keep energy active in the participants, and thus keep the scene going. The top penetrates the bottom with a tendril of hir energy, which then draws the bottom's energy out and into the top (See Brennan 1987, Belanger 2004). This energy then passes back into the bottom. The top may use physical contact to focus the tendril - s/he touches the bottom, using that touch to penetrate hir energetic body. The top can then draw on the bottom's energy. If the top doesn't replace most of the energy taken, s/he can effectively render any resistant bottom passive very quickly. This can turn energy work into a unique — but effective — form of bondage.

Other stimuli can also facilitate the draining. During any sort of play, whether it's painful or sensual, energy is raised; however, the top may modify those stimuli so that instead of just raising the normal amount of energy, they also drain extra energy from the bottom with each physical contact. The top directs the energy into the chosen purpose or goal. The bottom then ends up being a sort of energetic battery to power the magic. Additionally, the top can maintain complete control of the situation while the bottom is free to abandon hirself to the experience, thereby avoiding any inhibitions or other conscious thoughts that may adversely affect the outcome of the ritual.

While energetic draining can be a fun technique to use, it's also important to know how to return energy back to the bottom. In a case where energy is merely taken away but is not used for any magical purpose, Chia suggests the following: "The safeguard against this is the circulation of the energy through both partners' bodies. This exchange of energy eliminates the possibility that one partner will gain energy while the other one loses" (Chia 2005, p. 215). To circulate energy back into the bottom, the top simply returns it by sending it back through the tendril. Alternately, the bottom may learn how to work with energy hirself, so if necessary, s/he can simply take it back when the time is right. If any energy has been used for a magical working, then grounding, eating food, and a good night's rest should replenish that energy.

A gentler alternative to energetic draining is based on pore breathing and energy accumulation as described by Franz Bardon. Pore breathing works on the idea that a person's entire body breathes air through the pores of the body, drawing in ambient energy. "By breathing through the lungs and pores of your body, you inhale vital energy. With the power of your imagination, press this vital energy into your whole body to the point that it radiates dynamically. At this point your body should be like a luminous power, a focal point or burning point" (Bardon 1999, p. 111). Pore breathing is easy to do. Sit down and inhale through your nose. With each breath, try to focus on a part of your body, such as a finger, and pull the energy around the finger into it with your breath. With each exhale, the energy may go out, but as you practice this technique, you'll learn to retain the energy for longer periods. This energy can be stored and then used.

Bardon also points out that while pore breathing, you can draw in and accumulate specific elemental energy, which he usually associates with colors and sensations. For example, fire energy is red and hot, while air is warm and moist (Bardon 1999). Taylor uses the accumulation technique to draw in fiery energy, and then puts his finger on Lupa's skin while projecting the energy. She feels burned by it, even though no physical burns are left. This is an effective way to incorporate elements of fire play without lasting physical effects. Other elements may be utilized for their own particular effects.

The accumulative energy doesn't have to be strictly elemental in nature. Another variety of energy work as bondage is "sticky" energy. The top accumulates a handful of energy that has the qualities of something sticky, such as glue or sap. S/he then spreads it on the hands of the bottom, and "sticks" hir to a flat surface, such as a wall (Kaldera, 2006). As a psychological accompaniment, the top can tell the bottom that s/he can't move hir hands from the wall; they may slide up and down, but can't be removed entirely. Lupa has found that the combination of the energy work and the psychological triggers resembles a form of mild hypnosis; while she rationally knows that she could pull her hands away any time, she realizes, in this particular ASC, that this is a futile exercise. It's similar to bottoms and submissives that will hold a particular posture without moving when ordered, except with energy work added in. In fact, this "sticky" energy is useful in training a bottom or slave to hold a pose, by "sticking" hir body in place.

Bardon's energy techniques also provide an effective approach to breaking down a person's defensive shields without harming them. Pore breathing can open a person up, which is where the second approach to energy draining comes in. Instead of drawing energy into his own pores, Taylor will push his energy into Lupa's pores to infuse her with his energy. He breathes on her and uses the breath to convey the energy into her. While this technique can leave the opening party feeling very vulnerable, it can also be a very pleasurable experience, and one that isn't as forceful as the first one we described. One of our favorite variations on this technique is sharing breath -- kissing, but putting energy in the kiss so that the energy of both people swirls together.

Pore breathing can create a vortex of energy that cycles back and forth between the participants. This cycling creates an ASC, as both people feel drawn into each other more and more, and focus is narrowed down to the ritual itself. It's not unusual to see the other person's face change shape and color as the energy builds and affects the perception of the participants.

Taoist techniques are the third system we like to use. These techniques are handy for building energy vortexes, but don't involve breaking down energetic shields. During sex, one partner directs the energy through hirself to the other person, who then directs it back. The tongue is placed on the roof of the mouth to complete the energetic circuit. The energy is merged together and shared between the partners, again with the vortex result occurring. This approach doesn't involve any draining, but is useful for magical purposes. The energy cycles through each person, and when climax is reached, can be pushed toward the chosen practical goal. Alternately, you can focus the cycling energy to enhance the natural health of the body. This is what we usually use the energy vortex for. When one of us isn't feeling well, or if we just happen to be doing this technique, the cycling of the energy can be a very rejuvenating experience. We both feel energized after this energetic sexual practice.

Kink magic is a great way to charge magical items, particularly those aimed at love/lust magic (within reasonable limits, of course). However, the intent can be changed depending on the type of kink used. For example, forced feminization whose target is a budding male-to-female transgendered person may raise energy that can then be placed into a magical item to help enhance her comfort with herself as a woman. A collar or other symbol of a D/S relationship can be ritually charged through enchantment to strengthen the bond.

Previously enchanted items may also be brought into a kink magic scene. Dripping wax from a charged candle can imbue the bottom with the qualities of that candle. A dominant might do a private ritual before a scene to place a binding into a collar or cuffs. The accumulation of elemental energy a la Franz Bardon could be transferred to various tools and toys; a pinwheel could be charged with fire energy, for example.

Taylor Speaks:

I incorporate energy work into my sex life and kink scenes. In the very first scene I had with Lupa, I used energy work to top her. At first, she fought me, to the point that it was hard for me to enjoy the scene with her. I like it when a bottom fights, but the first time I scene with a person, I want hir to allow me to get to know hir. I want time to explore the person in-depth, to get a sense of how they react to my methods, and to tease them just enough to make sure they want to come back for more.

Because Lupa was struggling so much, I decided to do some energy work with her to put her into a more passive state while I got to know her reactions better. First, I drained her of some excess energy. This involved creating a tendril and using it to vamp energy

147

from her. I didn't take all of her energy, but I took enough to slow her down some. Once she was more passive, I chose to pore breathe the energy back into her. While I massaged her body, I began pore breathing. The soft sighs and surprised exclamations from her were gratifying to hear, because I could tell she really enjoyed the sensation of having energy breathed back into her.

After I finished the pore breathing and massage, I gently ran my fingers over her body. I extended energy into my fingers so she could feel my energy as it interacted with hers. At the same time, I called on the spirit of Fox, with which I resonate strongly, and asked it to help sooth and heal her further. I say "heal" because it was my first scene with her, and I noticed she was tense and in a bit of pain. My energy work wasn't just for pacifying her, but was focused also on healing. By the end of the night, she was a very happy, relaxed Lupa. (She later told me that she'd gained experience points from it.)

Lupa Speaks:

I'd never had anyone use energy work on me in a sexual context prior to Taylor, so this was a new experience for me! I'm normally a tough bottom, especially early on in a relationship. I don't like making it easy for someone to top me; it's just a dynamic that I prefer. It can take months and dozens of scenes to get me to be more cooperative; there's a lot of trust involved, and the tough bottom role is admittedly partly a defense mechanism (but also something that I enjoy for its own sake).

It was a surprise when he started calming me with energy; I was already more pliable by the time I noticed what had happened. I'm sensitive to energy in general, but he was very subtle. He tamed me without my realizing it was happening. Then there was the fun of putting that energy back in; Taylor is wonderfully sensual, and he made it incredibly relaxing and exciting all at once.

This scene introduced a trend in our relationship right from the beginning -- not only did Taylor introduce me to a new form of kink, he also taught me about a level of trust and intimacy that was new to me. Through the medium of energy, he was able to communicate to me a connection I had never achieved before, and showed me that it was safe for me to allow myself to be that vulnerable to him.

Final Thoughts

These are just a few examples of how you can incorporate practical magic into your kink rituals; feel free to modify them however you like. While the ASCs involved are often reserved for the functions of "high," or metamorphic, magic (which we'll discuss in the next chapter), it's possible to address everyday issues with them as well. After all, working on ascension is no good if your everyday life is a mess! Additionally, the magic involved can be used for otherwise non-magical kinky play, such as energetic bondage — we all like to just play sometimes.

Chapter Ten: Metamorphic Magic

Metamorphic magic is magic done for self-transformation and conscious evolution, and is primarily focused on a person's internal reality. It operates on the principle that shaping the microcosm also affects the macrocosm (and vice versa), creating more possibilities. This form of magic can be work intensive, with emotional and mental reprogramming occurring. It can be done on a solitary basis, but we find that the environment of kink is highly useful for drawing out the issues that need to be addressed. The goal is to put a person into an ASC using kink techniques where s/he can then address hir issues and change hir internal reality as needed. This type of magic can also involve connecting with external beings, such as deities, to learn from them or adopt their traits, either temporarily or permanently.

Facing and confronting inner demons and old issues is incredibly empowering. There is a release and a feeling of moving past obstacles. For many magicians, it's also a flexible approach to concepts of identity. The ability to change who you are to meet a particular situation is a realization that identity isn't set in stone, but can be related to how you perceive the world – and how the world perceives you.

Invocation, Mindfuck, and Roleplaying

The three elements of invocation, mindfuck, and roleplaying weave nicely together. In order to mindfuck someone or participate in believable roleplay, you have to be able to invoke an energy or personality other than your own. Some of the tools used in successful invocation call on the same imagination and suspension of disbelief as mindfuck and roleplaying.

The mindfuck is defined as "a scene tailored by the dominant with the intent of making it look more dangerous or edgy than it really is" (Warren 2000, p. 89). Mindfuck may include physical forms of edgeplay to heighten the drama, or it may be done empty-handed, with the only tools being the voice and the top's knowledge of the bottom's weak spots. It can involve pushing psychological buttons that unveil repressed emotional issues. Initially this may not seem terrifying, but imagine having your deepest parts suddenly exposed to the light of day -- things that even you have trouble facing, suddenly revealed for the top to play with. This can create an incredible sense of helplessness and vulnerability in a very short time, and toss the bottom into a deep headspace.

Roleplaying isn't as intense as mindfuck, but involves a similar suspension of disbelief. "Essential ingredients for any role-play scenario would be some degree of sensitivity about the role, or a true perception of the role about to be enacted, and the aura of sincerity and authenticity that you create" (Varrin 2004, p. 184). Skilled roleplaying has everyone believing, for the duration of the scene, that what they are doing is real. In addition to changes in posture and voice, elaborate additions, such as costumes and props, may add to the overall feel of the ritual.

Donning a maid outfit and pretending that the master or mistress of the house punishes the maid for sloppy work is a clichéd example of roleplay, something adopted playfully to provoke a response and playact a certain power exchange. Pretending to be a maid isn't just a change in roles; for some people, it involves accessing a persona other than the one used everyday. Such changes add spice to a scene or make a person feel vulnerable by taking on a risqué role that s/he would not normally adopt. Roleplay is usually for fun, though it can be an incredibly useful psychological tool.

This is partly because roleplay involves your level of comfort with who you perceive yourself to be. A person who is comfortable with hirself can change hirself as needed, fitting any role and playing any part, because s/he is confident in hir preferred identity and hir ability to return to it at any time. Forced crossdressing, particularly involving the emasculation of men, can be a way to challenge the bottom's sense of self and help hir learn to access other personality aspects.

Because many scenes already involve roleplaying to some extent, it's not hard for the top or bottom to go to the next level -- invocation. Roleplaying is a game of make-believe, pretending to be something you aren't. That persona is like a costume that's put on and taken off. Invocation, on the other hand, involves allowing another entity (or alternate aspect of the self) to temporarily share or possess your body, while retaining some conscious awareness and control of your primary sense of self. Invocation is a blending of your personality with that of the entity/aspect you've invoked. Invocation, in this context, is sometimes referred to as channeling and involves allowing the entity to become you temporarily, in order to switch the scene into a ritual (Easton & Hardy 2001). Channeling involves the assumption of a role and a willingness to allow the deity a chance to share the sensations you are experiencing. It also allows you to establish boundaries and show physical limitations for subsequent invocations of the entity. Your body's muscle memories, and the hardwiring of your brain, all form parameters that the entity must work within. While the entity has some level of control over the actions, so do you.

However, this form of invocation isn't as potent as possession. When most people think of possession, they usually think of the movie *The Exorcist*, in which a malevolent spirit controlled a character. These Hollywood stereotypes about possession are highly inaccurate. A person's head will not spin like a barstool, and you are in little danger of possession by an "evil spirit" that will cause trouble while in your body.

Voodoo may also come to mind, where the *loa* temporarily possess the faithful in order to experience the physical world for a time. In religions where possession most often occurs, other people carefully monitor the act to make sure no one comes to harm. The possession involves a complete takeover by the entity, with the personality of the person receding to a subconscious level. This means that the entity has full control of the body and the resultant actions. The possessed person may or may not remember what occurred while s/he was possessed, and it is usually up to the entity whether that person will have access to those memories.

In some possession-based religions, it's assumed that the person is being ridden like a horse, and so doesn't necessarily have as much of a choice as one might think. Additionally, any harm done during the possession is usually attributed to the entity, not the person who owns the body. This is why it's important for others to monitor the situation. Possession is one of the most intense ways of working with an entity, and it can shock your system if you've never been exposed to the idea of invocation before; for this reason, it's probably a good idea not to work with possession if you're brand new to magic.

Taylor has experienced full possession. One pop culture entity he has worked with is Thiede, from the *Wraeththu* series by Storm Constantine. Taylor has a strong connection to this entity, and will occasionally allow it full possession of his body so it can interact with the world. When this occurs, Taylor isn't consciously aware of what's happening and usually has no memory of the incident. Lupa has noticed that his features and ways of speaking and moving change. We haven't used this type of invocation often in our kink magic practices, mainly because we find it to be risky.

Lupa once energetically opened Taylor and inadvertently invoked a hostile entity into him. It didn't hurt her or Taylor, but it didn't want to leave his body. She had to banish it. The only other time we've done such an invocation was when the person doing the invocation was bound and couldn't move much. In such a situation it's still important to keep an eye on the person being possessed to avoid accidental injury. We suggest that you take care with using a full possession invocation in kink magic, as the entity you are dealing with is not the person you would otherwise play with. The entity will not necessarily respect the usual boundaries.

There is the question of responsibility, specifically with regard to possession. For example, in Voodoo, when the *loa* decide to ride someone, anything that happens to that body is attributed to the *loa*, not the person. However, there are people on hand who know how to work with the *loa* when they incarnate temporarily; it's not a matter of these spirits running amok using their believers' bodies. We have, however, seen cases in the pagan and occult communities in which people have done some really stupid and/or destructive things while supposedly working with invocation or possession, and then blaming those actions on the invoked entity. The problem with this is that it can't be proven, especially in a court of law. If you invoke Thor and then go smash someone's head in with a hammer, you're the one who's going to take the blame for it. The same goes for kink magic: if you invoke an entity, and then violate the consensual boundaries of the ritual, it's on your head.

The moral of the story? Know who and what you're invoking, and have people nearby who can help if things get out of hand. Truth be told, we think that most instances of people blaming invoked entities were nothing more than people letting their ids run free, and trying to pass it off as magic. Not only does this get people in trouble, but it looks bad for the magical community in general. If you have never done an invocation before, we highly recommend reading basic techniques and trying them out before working with the rest of the material on the subject in this book.

As for us, Taylor utilizes both forms of invocation while Lupa prefers only partial invocation. You can invoke whatever you feel is most appropriate for your workings, whether that includes deities, totems, devas, or whatever entities you feel comfortable with. Taylor invokes mostly pop culture entities, with the occasional traditional entity thrown in when needed, while Lupa prefers to work with her totem spirits and various personality aspects.

We mentioned earlier that sometimes invocation can involve an aspect of self, rather than an external entity. Taylor invokes his dominant aspect by drawing on the emotions he associates with that side. These emotions include anger and aggression, but can also include the need for control, fear, stress, etc. Most of the emotions are considered "negative," though this doesn't mean his use of them is negative. Indeed, in many ways kink can be a healthy way of venting emotions and stress. In taking on his dominant aspect, Taylor can freely express these emotions in a controlled manner, and integrate that control back into his usual self. By temporarily isolating certain emotions and behaviors and personifying them, it's possible to gain a greater and clearer understanding of them than if they're mixed into the general soup of the self.

This type of invocation is called aspecting and more people do it than they realize. We all act differently when we're around specific people. You probably act, speak and maybe even dress differently when you're around your parents than when you're at a dungeon or play party (If not, you must have some very open-minded parents!). In either case, you're accessing a unique aspect of yourself tailored to a particular setting and choice of company. The benefit of aspecting is that you can use it to develop yourself more fully as an individual, adding to the possibilities of who you are.

One of Lupa's more extreme experiments with aspecting involved temporarily dividing herself into four different personae, buying each one a separate wardrobe, and living each day entirely as a different aspect. The clothing acted as an anchor that when worn, invoked the desired aspect and triggered the specific behavior and thoughts patterns of that persona.

The disadvantage to this approach is that if you take it too far, it can lead to identity issues, with an aspect wanting to split off to become its open separate personality. At that point, the aspect has to be reintegrated into the overall personality, which means that the long-term invocation should stop and some internal work, such as meditation, should be used to begin the integration. The integration may take some time, but once it's done, the person will actually be more balanced because s/he will have incorporated the previously undeveloped attributes into the core personality. For example, Lupa's initial experiment was six weeks long, but the residual effects involving one particular aspect lasted for well over a year afterward.

Some of our aspecting work deals with gender identity. Part of the reason Lupa did her four-aspect experiment was to explore the parts of herself that identified as male (not just masculine) and to integrate them into herself, exploring the idea of the androgynous gender. Since gender is how we mentally think of ourselves, it's not a physical change, but it *is* a change in how we identify ourselves.

Gender may be expressed throughcrossdressing. There is an important difference between people who cross-dress for fetish reasons, and people who cross-dress because they genuinely feel that their gender is the opposite of the body they inhabit. In the former case, a fetish cross-dresser enjoys dressing up in clothes associated with the opposite sex as a sexual thrill. In the latter case, s/he may feel a sense of gender dysphoria or discomfort with the physical body. This feeling prompts hir to change the outward appearance as much as possible. For example, a person who has female genitalia, but identifies as male, will dress in masculine, baggy clothing to hide the curves he has. Some transition their physical sex to the sex that they feel is most appropriate to them.

In kink magic, you can usecrossdressing for invocation of god-forms that don't fit the usual gender perception of the person. A man can cross-dress to invoke a goddess, and vice versa. This can give the person a different gender identity as well as providing a better medium for the godform to use.

"Forced"crossdressing is used as a humiliation technique, but may also be utilized in resolving internal issues regarding one's identity. One example is provided below.

Taylor Speaks:

Lupa tends to identify as androgynous or fairly masculine. Once, as I was topping her, I thought I might have some fun with her gender identity by force-feminizing her. When she identifies as male, Lupa lowers her voice and dresses as masculine as possible. She also tends to shy away from anything even remotely feminine. On the day I force feminized her, she'd identified as male and so didn't expect when I made her dress like a woman. The shock she experienced in being force feminized proved very useful for putting her into a deep subspace.

First, I made her pull out her hair band, so her hair was unbound. Then I ordered her to get a feminine dress. I rejected several of her choices until she picked out a frilly white dress. I told her to put it on. At first she resisted, but I grabbed her hair and insisted on it. She reluctantly put the dress on and I marched her into the bathroom and asked her how she felt. She said she didn't

156

like it, that it didn't feel like her. I then made her put on some cosmetics and asked her again how she felt. She still said it didn't feel like her.

What stood out to me about the experience was when she was in a dress, she really did look out of her element. Being force feminized was good for her because it forced her to confront an aspect of herself she normally avoided. We spent quite a bit of that afternoon talking afterwards about the scene and how she felt about her femininity.

I could use this forcedcrossdressing in the opposite manner, to produce discomfort with the overall appearance, and then using that discomfort as a form of invocation for a particular godform -- or even for the archetypal consciousness associated with a particular gender. Lupa did just such a working with me.

Lupa Speaks:

The tables had turned. I was feeling particularly sadistic one day while topping him, though I don't recall what prompted me to express it in this way. While Taylor tends to be less genderfluid than I am, staying more or less androgynous rather than oscillating back and forth between male and female, I wanted to bring out that which was *negatively* stereotypically feminine in him—vulnerability, weakness, objectification.

At an earlier date, I had bought him a long black broomstick skirt at a pagan gathering. One of the joys of the festival atmosphere is that people can wear whatever they want, and those skirts are comfortable. I made him put it on, then ordered him into the bedroom for an impromptu rape scene.

Rape isn't about sex—it's about control. I allowed the part of me that must have control over everything to surface, and I called on the archetype of the rapist, the person (not always male) who takes what s/he wants through sex. I blindfolded him, and put Chapstick on him, telling him it was lipstick so he'd be pretty for me. Then I grabbed him, touched and groped him all over, lifted his skirt and whipped him. In short, I evoked in him the terror a rape victim feels, the vulnerability of wearing a skirt that leaves little protection for a vulnerable area, and the violation of personal space.

The crossdressing served to shake him out of his comfort zone. Spiritual androgyne though he may be, he still has a male body, and there are certain social parameters that come with that. While men can certainly be victims of sexual assault, there is a social vulnerability that comes part and parcel with the perception of being female in American culture. I wanted to impart on him, for just a while, the feeling of discomfort and fear that a person in a female body (genetic or not) often feels when catcalled, groped, assaulted or otherwise violated. It worked — it threw him into a deep subspace, and opened him up to what I had evoked.

We played like that for a while, and allowed it to be a cathartic experience. I felt that he had a better idea of some of the fear and vulnerability women can feel on a regular basis (though he was previously aware of it). It also allowed me to explore some of my own feelings of vulnerability, as well as explore the headspace of the kind of person who evokes that fear.

Pathworking

Pathworking uses visualization to create a mental space where you can work with certain internal issues, meet with an entity to obtain information, or otherwise explore unordinary realms. An excellent example of pathworking is visualizing a large dining hall with different doorways. Each one leads to a specific aspect of your personality or interaction with other people. For example, the door behind where you sit at the imagined dinner table might be the door that represents your mate or your higher self, and opening that door allows you to interact with that person or aspect within a controlled setting (Farrell 2004). Pathworking is well-known among occult Kabbalists, who use the Tree of Life as a map to evolution of the self. Any magical paradigm or system may apply the practice of pathworking, the symbols and entities within acting as guides along the way. In some cases, another person may guide the pathworking by reading a script or telling a story. Others are entirely personal and are free-form.

We enjoy combining pathworking and sex magic, using sex as a way of acting out a journey — and we're not alone. For example, Ashcroft-Nowicki uses the sephiroth on the Kabbalistic Tree of Life for the sex magic pathworking. Her model works well, though it is limited by focusing on the sephiroth alone as opposed to incorporating the twenty two paths that connect the sephiroth to each other. Including the paths with the sephiroth would make for a lot of sex magic and pathworking, but it is an effective way of learning the various correspondences to the tree of life (and will certainly keep you busy!). Incorporating pathworking into sex magic makes it easy to learn about a particular subject when you physically act out and mentally explore that subject, during and after the act of sex. Sex is an excellent imprinter because it leaves each person open; it can be a vulnerable act for that same reason. Thus, you should only do these workings with people you trust.

Pathworking works well with kink magic, because there are techniques and approaches in kink that set up conditions similar to pathworking. In one sense, kink is about telling a story, setting up a scene and believing in the reality that the scene is attempting to create. In a scene, this is accomplished through mindfuck and roleplaying, and through use of different tools and props, all of which serve to create the suspension of disbelief that makes a scene so powerful.

It is important to remember that pathworking is on one level a reality, but it is also a fantasy, allowing us to explore our deepest layers of emotion and consciousness. You must still be careful. "The fantasy frame can help both partners enter freely into the spirit of the working, and can also mark it out more sharply in your minds: this is a play, a special activity, which adds to but does not supplant other kinds of workings. Psychological frames such as these can unearth serious issues around control and surrender" (Williams 1990, p. 110). Pathworking is one way of exploring these psychological frames, by enabling us to journey into ourselves and deal with past issues or emergent desires in a safe and healthy manner. It's important to remember that as people explore and are guided, there will be times when the ritual may need to stop. If this happens, stop and resume later, when you and your partner(s) are ready to travel down that particular path again. You don't want to force yourself or anyone else into territory you don't feel ready to explore; this is counterproductive and can create even more psychological wounds.

There are two distinct, but complementary, primary roles in pathworking:

> The journeyer is going to be pierced or whipped or otherwise done to, but for their own purposes, essentially to prepare for a more or less solo journey. So the ritual is about the bottom, for the bottom's use and purposes. The top, the person who does the piercing or tying up or whatever, is not so much dominant as guide, priest, support person. (Easton & Hardy 2004, p. 189)

159

Pathworking this way is intense. The bottom's body and mind are fully engaged. We disagree however, that the ritual is only about the bottom. Too often in BDSM culture, the emphasis is only on this role; however, the top is an invaluable part of the scene and the ritual. Without the top, the bottom cannot journey. Sometimes the journey is as much about the top as it is about the bottom; they share the ritual journey. The experience is different for each participant, but each journey somewhere, learn something, and offer comfort to each other. All participants in a ritual play equal roles, and all are equally responsible for each other. This includes the point at which the ritual dissolves the boundaries of the participants, opening a path for both the bottom and the top to explore. The top is a guide, and yet the bottom also guides, revealing through hir pain and other sensations if the top is on the right path.

In another sense the connection created through pathworking is an alchemical one, "In Carnal Alchemy the dominant takes the role of the alchemist, while the submissive is the very substance being transformed – to begin with perhaps 'lead,' but at the end of the process the purest 'gold.' Magically speaking the working of submissive Carnal Alchemy is most effective when you are trying to change things about yourself" (Dawn & Flowers 2001, p. 32). Dawn and Flowers later point out that the top is not just changing the inner reality of the bottom, but also hir own reality, projecting onto the bottom the changes that s/he needs for hirself. The working changes both, because both participate in a ritual that changes their internal realities. This rings true with Taoist sexual alchemy and other forms of Western sex magic, where the sex is used as an agent of transformation for both partners (Frantzis 2001b, Williams 1990, U.D. 2001). Kink magic, in general, runs with this idea. It's not just about the bottom, but also about the top; while some rituals may favor one or the other, there's room for both overall.

Taylor Speaks:

For the majority of our scenes, I tend to be the top. As such, I've played the role of the guide, opening Lupa and taking her into meditations where she interacts with other beings. Sometimes these pathworkings can be intense for me, especially with what I do to her to push her triggers and help her face past issues. After the workings are over, sometimes I need the comfort or care more than

160

she does, because the full weight of my actions hits me, inspiring guilt. Rationally, I know she's thankful for the experience, and wanted it, but emotionally, the idea that I have hurt her or caused her to recall old wounds can powerfully affect me.

A vivid example: I once invoked her past partners, including one partner in particular who'd been abusive to her. I acted just like hir, treating Lupa like an object, telling her what a good fuck she was, and then walking away. She cried, and couldn't move, looking terrified and defeated. The kicker was when I leaned on her like a piece of furniture, turned on the Playstation 2, and pretended to start playing. She gave a growl, rolled out from under me, grabbed my hair and started to hit me. I told her, "Lupa, it's Taylor!" She stopped, snapped out of her ASC, and cried for a few moments, but managed to pull herself together. The scene was over -- and then I started crying. I felt horrible. Sure, she needed this experience and it helped her heal some wounds, but I still felt horrible for opening those wounds. Instead of me comforting her, she comforted me. In this case, the bottom was responsible for the top.

Lupa Speaks:

This was a rough one to go through. I've mostly had healthy relationships, but there are a couple of exceptions. There was one in particular that really stuck with me -- I was stuck with all the housework and responsibilities, while the other person spent a lot of hir free time playing video games and other frivolous things. In retrospect, there was much more wrong with that relationship, on my end as well as hirs, but that particular slice of negativity had seriously impacted me.

I *hate* being objectified. The only time I've ever allowed it in play was the human altar ritual we discuss in Chapter 12. No playing footstool, or ashtray, or anything else that's dehumanizing; it's just NMK. This particular instance was prior to the human altar ritual, so I was even less open to the idea. When Taylor started tearing into me about how I was a good fuck, it really upset me. But when he had the audacity to treat me like a piece of furniture, I'd had enough.

I'm a fan of being a difficult bottom when the situation presents itself. However, I don't actually try to harm the top; I just struggle, and maybe shove and nip a little. But this situation pushed me way too far, and I was seriously out for blood. (This, by the way, is a classic example of what can go wrong in a psychology-heavy ritual.)

Fortunately, Taylor is much larger and stronger than I am, so he was able to protect himself. But it took him actually speaking to me, and reminding me that I was with him, and not my ex, to wake me up. It didn't take long to come out of ASC, mainly because the attack in and of itself had been sufficiently cathartic, so I had a quick recovery.

Taylor, on the other hand, wasn't so lucky. He has a hard time when we have everyday disagreements over little things and the conversation gets heated—he just doesn't like the idea of harming me in any way. It was no surprise when, after acting out that sort of psychological abuse, he collapsed in tears. (We told you these things can be hard on the top, too!) I was able to help him pull himself together, but it took gentle words, reassurance, and patience on my part.

Practical Pathworking

Now that you know the theoretical dynamics, it's time to explore the practical aspects of pathworking. You don't necessarily have to make it cathartic for everyone, but you definitely want to focus on working through a particular issue as thoroughly as possible without going so far as to cause more harm than good. This should involve discussion before the scene even occurs. For instance, what type of issue will be explored? Will it be spiritual, emotional, relationship, or another kind of issue? Who does it focus on?

Once you've determined your issue, it's possible to create a scene around it. As an example, once we know the issue that the bottom wants to deal with, the top will consider what type of pathworking should be constructed, as well as how to hit the bottom's relevant triggers so that s/he can benefit from the pathworking, while at the same time not pushing hir to use the safe word/action.

However, sometimes a person can only make so much progress on a painful issue. If multiple pathworking sessions for the issue are needed, then go with that format. We find that it's best to allow an organic flow to pathworking, i.e. we don't follow a specific format, but improvise as needed. Some people will follow scripts, but a scene is a dynamic arena and following a script may not be as beneficial in such a setting. If your first ritual doesn't entirely exorcise the demon, so to speak, you can use its progress to design the next one.

We delay the actual ritual for several days after we've discussed what needs to be done. This gives the top some time to find inspiration, as well as heightens the bottom's anticipation. We won't immediately start the actual pathworking when the time for the ritual comes, either. Instead, it's better to get the bottom into a mild subspace, where s/he can still respond and move, but s/he is into the scene. At that point, a verbal/visual cue is useful for triggering the bottom's issue. This cue could be an action that triggers a memory, such as a slap across the face, or a specific phrase that brings a memory to the surface.

Alternately, if the bottom is journeying alone, the trigger could consist of the top opening the bottom energetically while assuming the role of the guide. The top then proceeds to push the bottom further into subspace with hir actions, while questioning or otherwise guiding the bottom, or simply allowing hir to explore on hir own.

Energy Work in Pathworking

We often use energy work in this context to help with emotional healing. Emotion equals energy in motion. Even an energetic blockage is energy that is in motion, albeit a motion that turns in on itself and hardens the energy to create a feeling of dis-ease. It should be no surprise that emotions are linked to our overall health. Stress, unhappiness, anger, and other such emotions can, if improperly handled, lead to physical complications including ulcers, headaches, and hypertension, while also weakening the immune system, thereby increasing the risk of illness.

BDSM is one of our stress-relievers. By having an outlet where we can express pent-up stress, we are able to vent emotions, circulate energy, and have a satisfying experience. BDSM doesn't take the place of communication, and our rule is to never take our anger out at each other during a scene. Instead, we talk about it, give each other space, and/or vent it in ways that aren't harmful to other people. We may deal with the residual internal issues later in a pathworking ritual, but we never bring genuine anger into the bedroom.

Some emotions are repressed for so long and have created such a blockage that they can only be dealt with in a pathworking, either in a kink ritual or in solo practice. When working alone, deep meditation can be useful for gradually dissolving the blockage and working through the corresponding emotions, memories, and related feelings that occur as a result of the dissolution. Individual practice can also be used in conjunction with kink magic. Taylor, for example, actively worked on dissolving energetic blockages on his own, but kink magic pathworking sessions greatly aided the dissolution. Lupa was able to help him accelerate the process of dissolution by giving him situations where he could fully feel and process the emotional pain, while having her nearby to provide comfort, discipline, or anything else he needed.

In this context, the top uses energy work to find the blockage and pull it out of the bottom, while also handling the corresponding emotional damage. Below we present individual impressions and experiences with this process.

Lupa Speaks:

I really hadn't done much with energy work, beyond sensing energy, before I met Taylor. However, when involved with another magician, I enjoy trading notes and discovering what my partner likes to work with. Taylor's been working with energy since almost the beginning of his practice, so he's become quite good at it, and I've been picking up techniques throughout the course of our relationship.

I remember the first time I really put it to use, though. It was soon after we'd started dating, and he'd been working through issues with regard to previous relationships. While his most recent relationship had been wonderful for him, he's had negative experiences with other people over the years.

Memories of one former partner in particular had been bothering him, and he was having trouble deprogramming reactions to things that reminded him of her. Wishing to aid his suffering, I soft topped him to calm him and ease him into a more receptive mode. Then I drew forth my rarely-used jealousy in conjunction with the more lupine aspects of my nature. I invoked the aspect of myself that is the bitch-wolf incarnate -- the alpha bitch who will terrorize the rest of the females in the pack to be sure that she is the only one who breeds. Someone dared to harm my mate, and I was pissed off.

I channeled that rage into energetic claws on the ends of my fingers, part of a spiritual shift. Carefully, as not to cause Taylor any more pain than necessary, I symbolically opened up his chest with these claws, energetically revealing the root of the problem. There, buried deep within his chest, was a chunk of energy that to my mind's eye was a small red heart made of that cheap plastic that kid's water guns from the dollar store are made of. It sat next to his heart, but just as with any foreign body, it rankled and irritated the (energetic) flesh around it. The manifestation was appropriate, as the past situation involved false shows of love from his partner, and so the residual energy of this false love had shown up as a fake heart.

I excised the plastic heart and held it in my hands. I didn't want to casually discard the energy away where it might harm someone else. Instead, I decided to transform it. First, I willed it to become pure energy; in my mind's eye it became a pool of blood in my hands. Then I drank it down to show Taylor that it could no longer harm him. There remained a gaping hole in his energetic body where the plastic heart had been, so I took some of my own green-wolf energy and filled in the hole to protect it until it healed over time. Then I closed up his chest again, healing the wounds, calling upon the archetype of Lupa, the wolf-mother, to soothe the aches and pains.

The ritual was a success; Taylor showed immediate signs of improvement, and although there've been occasional relapses, the memories and the residual energy no longer have the impact they once did.

Taylor Speaks:

When I act as a guide for a spiritual journey, I don't necessarily assume the role of an entity or deity. My persona does change, however. I'm harsher and more demanding, pushing Lupa past her threshold, while at the same time keeping her from using the safe word. This can involve changing tactics when she least expects it. For instance, I'll start with physical punishment and then when she adjusts to that, I'll switch to psychological button pushing, or I'll move from a sensuous massage to a sudden hard slap. Occasionally, I'll even make her temporarily top me. The purpose of all this is to push her in directions she doesn't expect, while eliciting reactions that indicate she's going into an ASC conducive for the work involved.

One approach we've both found useful is integrating energy work into the pathworking. I imagine that my fingers become claws or knives that can open up the shields she has around her, allowing me to pull out any energy that doesn't belong. Similar to what Lupa does with me, I'll place my fingers on her chest and draw a straight line to her belly. I'll then make several other horizontal energetic slits on the sides of the vertical slit. At that point, her energetic body will be opened up.

When the energetic body is opened, Lupa usually gasps in surprise. There can be feelings of cold, heat, or tingly sensations, and a sense of vulnerability because the inner energetic organs are exposed. Lupa usually experiences sensations of limited movement, probably due to the shock. I experience these same symptoms when she opens me up.

Once I've opened Lupa, I'll either remove the harmful energy or evoke the specific psychological trigger that will bring that energy to the surface. The energy often appears as a brown/black sludge, representing her emotional pain and trauma. I'll scoop it out of her, then transmute it into energy I can release into the environment, where it can be recycled. During this, I'll comfort her, or if needed, say things I know will evoke the emotions and experiences that need to be unblocked.

In one instance, I pushed Lupa's triggers about her selfishness by detailing to her how she was selfish and had hurt others. Hearing this hurt her, but it was useful for drawing the emotions to the surface and allowing her to find peace with the selfishness issue. Through the energetic working, we were able to remove or evolve her associated negative feelings and help her attain balance, aiding her in communicating her need for space and alone time to other people. At the same time, she learned how to make time for other people so that they didn't feel left out of her life.

Once the energetic healing has occurred, it's important to stitch the surgical incision back up. I'll apply healing energy to replace the stagnant energy. Then I'll run my hands over the energetic cuts, sealing them and reestablishing the defenses of the energetic body.

Energy work, when combined with pathworking, is a useful medium of communication. As the two examples above show, energy work can strip away the defenses, revealing the soft underbelly of the beast. It also aids in deprogramming specific learned behaviors that cause us to *react* as opposed to consciously *acting*. Once a person is free of reactions, the energy s/he has invested in those reactions is also free, no longer creating a blockage. That energy can then be directed toward healthier purposes.

Exorcising Demons

Old magical grimoires such as the Goetia depict scores of demons that the magician must control in order to compel them to aid. Certain demons are called to acquire wealth, love, knowledge, and other sought after valuables. Once a demon is evoked and has served its purpose, however, it must be banished to avoid having it wreak havoc on the magician's life.

Exorcism is sometimes needed when you have a particularly stubborn demon. While the rarely-seen but often-fictionalized Catholic version is the best known, various magical systems have their own methods of ridding a person of both literal and metaphorical demons. One evening Lupa decided to create a variant on this idea.

Lupa Speaks:

Taylor was troubled by fallout from an issue that had raised its ugly head a few months prior. Now, it's our general policy to deal with things to the best of our ability - and then let them drop. Once a situation is either resolved or unsalvageable, we prefer to let it wind down on its own, feeding it as little as possible. Still, we are only human, and occasionally something will get under one or the other person's skin and rankle there a while. This usually results in a banishing ritual of one flavor or another.

First, I took Taylor by his collar and led him into the bedroom, then began to brush his hair to get him into a more submissive mindset. Once he had hit a nice light sub space, I clipped a leash to his collar, made him crouch down on the bed with his back exposed, and slapped him across the shoulders with a flogger to get his attention.

Then came the fun part.

Still using the leash to hold him down, I grabbed his hair to hold his ear close to my mouth as I whispered:

By the collar you wear
By the silver sigils around your neck
By my mark upon your chest
By the power I have over you

I bind you, Taylor Ellwood
My will is yours, and you will do as I command
By my friends, family and guardians
Who shall strike you down if you disobey!

As I chanted this, I called forth the figurative demon that had plagued him with worry, and it burst forth; his facial expression, posture, voice and energy shifted to a bestial, snarling, vengeful thing. He raged against his bonds, the collar and leash, but did me no harm.

Next, I commanded him to clean the mirror over the bed. I gave him a red lipstick and told him to draw a sigil representing each one of the sources of his worry on the mirror's surface. I made him kneel before the mirror with his hands against the wall, and had him project all his rage and negativity through the sigils on the mirror. The reflective surface used the sigils as a focus to bounce the emotions and energy back out towards the people and places that had originally caused Taylor his grief. To heighten the effect, I flogged him as he released this energy, adding to the purging purpose of the rite.

Once he had exhausted all of his rage, Taylor collapsed on the bed. I had him turn onto his stomach and began to rub lotion into his skin to help soothe the marks from the whip. As I did so, I banished the demon in a gentle voice:

I release you from this body where you no longer belong
I send you back to those who collectively created you
This is no longer your home; I bid you return to what now is your home
To those who created you.
I call upon the owner of this body, Taylor Ellwood
Your demon is gone; you no longer have need of it.

This served as an effective way to remove an unnecessary stressor in both of our lives, as neither one of us likes to see the other suffer (in a bad way). However, it was also a fascinating twist on a traditional form of magic. Most of the time, evocation and invocation are associated with external entities. However, in this case, the dual evocation/invocation involved a section of Taylor's energy, personified as a demon, and then banished back to the hellish people and situations that planted it in him in the first place.

Taylor Speaks:

When Lupa performed this exorcism of my personal demons by calling out the demon within me, I was still aware and in my body, if not fully in control. The one aspect of this working that stood out to me was how different my body felt and how different my face looked while I was expressing the demon. I felt as if I had a long bony tail, and I felt more muscular and feral. I imagined a kind of visceral stink rising from body. My chest felt as if it was on fire, my pain called forth in a way I couldn't deny feeling.

My face changed. It was much more angular and accentuated. My teeth formed a rictus grin and I felt as if the skin on my cheeks stretched tight over the muscle and bone. The noises that came from my mouth were animal-like grunts and mews.

Sometimes I'd try to resist Lupa when she commanded me, but always she was stronger than I was. I was bound by the collar to do her will. When she told me to express myself into the mirror, I could feel all of the negative energy, hurt and pain from the past leaving my body, taking the demon away as it gave voice and artistic expression to that which plagued us both. When we were finished with the ritual, I felt emptied of a pain I'd carried, and I slept very well that night.

Breaking and Rebuilding

The demons needn't be literal, however; nor will they necessarily be easily identifiable. One core issue we share is a fear of abandonment, and while Taylor was aware of his fear, it came out rather unexpectedly in Lupa. In one particular pathworking, Taylor tried to break her, putting her into a deep and vulnerable subspace so that she would know how it felt and be aware of the signs of a bottom reaching the breaking point. This would aid her in topping him or someone else without causing harm.

Taylor Speaks:

I invoked Albedo from the video game series *Xenosaga*; this entity was both a sadist and masochist, enjoying inflicting psychological and physical pain upon himself and others. I had a good impression of how the character spoke and acted, so to invoke the character, I adopted Albedo's accent and mannerisms, and the energy of my hands ended in claws similar to his.

I/Albedo knew what psychological buttons to push to break down Lupa's resistance. Rather than simply inflicting pain on her until she relented, we injured *my* body to emphasize her inability to stop us, making her feel even more helpless.

This pushed her to a point where she could no longer move or act on her own; she was effectively broken. I/Albedo then got up and walked out of the apartment, calling for her to come after us. The notion of being left in a broken state awoke the fear of abandonment in Lupa; already broken, she had no defenses against this particular inner demon. When she didn't come when called, I realized something was wrong and ended the invocation. I walked back in, banished Albedo, and held Lupa for a while, reassuring her. It took some time, but eventually I brought her out of subspace, grounded her, and talked with her over this newest discovery.

This pathworking helped Lupa not only become an effective top, focused more on the sensitivity of the bottom (she'd top me the very next day for the first time), but also made her consciously aware of her abandonment issues. She was then able to process the issue, instead of unconsciously letting it influence her behavior. We've since worked on banishing this particular demon in both of us in subsequent rituals

Lupa Speaks:

I had been hesitant to try topping Taylor when we first started playing together because I was worried I'd inadvertently harm him. I'd had no practical experience in being dominant in a kinky context, on either a scene-by-scene or lifestyle basis. I'd considered it, but I hadn't actually put my thoughts into practice.

Being broken in a scene was one of the best things to ever happen for my career as a switch. While I'd been pushed to helplessness in non-kinky situations, allowing someone to push me that far in a kink situation was a hard limit for me. This particular incident caught me off guard, though. We had been playing with each other for several months, so we were getting more comfortable with our scenes and tastes. Taylor had already taken me in some interesting directions, new territory for me.

I was caught unprepared when, at the climax of a particularly intense scene, he suddenly acted as if he was leaving. He put on his clothes, grabbed his car keys, and walked out the door. I think he expected me to follow him. However, I literally could not move. There wasn't anything wrong with my body (beyond the usual

170

bruises and other marks that are a natural byproduct of hard topping). It was all psychological. There I was, curled up in the center of the bed, released of all physical bondage—and I was paralyzed by the fear of abandonment.

No matter how well we think we may know ourselves, the deeper we dig into our psyches, the more surprises we may find. I never would have guessed that I had abandonment issues; unlike many other flaws I've worked through, there had never been any noticeable sign of this particular fear. But there was no doubt about it—Taylor and I had inadvertently uncovered something new.

Being the responsible person he is, intensely connected to me on numerous levels, he immediately sensed something was wrong when I failed to follow him out the door. He came back, banished the entity he'd invoked, and focused on making sure I was all right. As is our usual protocol, he calmed me down, and then let me talk. And I talked quite a bit, as I recall. There was so much to this particular fear. The more I examined it, the more I realized how subtly it had woven through my life throughout the years.

That part of me might have remained undiscovered if he hadn't broken me the way he had. He's done so several times since then, and each time I've been able to uncover additional destructive aspects of my psyche secretly ripping away at my subconscious, unnoticed and unchecked. It takes courage on both our parts, but it's worth pushing that boundary ever further.

As for topping, well, as Taylor mentioned, the next night was the first time I ever topped him. Being broken introduced me to one of the deepest levels accessible by a top. He showed me where I could push him—and how to do it in a careful manner. Overall, I believe my experience bottoming has helped to make me a better top, because I've seen the edge of my personal abyss, and seen where I could have toppled right in. Had Taylor left me lying there instead of coming back in, it would have taken a very long time for me to put myself back together again. Because I had that experience, I learned more about my responsibilities as a top. As a bottom, I have gained another way to explore my depths in a manner that allows me to create positive change in my personal microcosm.

A Different Twist on Metamorphic Magic and Kink

One question we've heard raised (including while we were writing this book) is, what happens if you end up burned out on kink—or sex in general?

Now, we're not professionally licensed sex therapists, so we're speaking solely from our own experiences as magicians. (Here, have a shaker of salt, just in case.) What we've noticed in our experiences and observations is that burnout from sex, kinky or otherwise, isn't so uncommon or abnormal as one might fear. People just don't like to talk about it, partly because there's such pressure in today's society to A) not talk about sex in any serious manner, and B) admit that you're not an absolutely perfect lover every single time.

The causes for burnout are numerous. Maybe you're bored, tired of the same old stuff. This is why we tend to throw in some vanilla sessions to keep us from getting too overloaded with the kink. We also like researching new toys and techniques to use on each other to keep our play from becoming too predictable. It's also why we maintain a polyfuckerous lifestyle; occasionally it's nice to play with someone else. After all, variety is the spice of life! (On the other hand, if you're currently in a monogamous relationship, this is not advice to go and find someone else to sleep with!)

Sometimes there's something more to it than boredom, though. What we've found is that stress is one of the most common libido-killers out there, whether you're no longer into kink, or not into anything sex-related at all. The stress itself can come from any of a number of sources, and not all of them are obvious.

For example, when we moved to Seattle, Lupa's libido took a plunge. It didn't disappear entirely, but things did get kind of rocky for a while. Thankfully, Taylor was patient enough to wait it out and help her figure out what the problem was. We figured out pretty quickly that it wasn't just a case of boredom, and finally determined that it was a combination of internal and external stress points. These ranged from employment dissatisfaction to being stuck in a too-large city, as well as a lot of internal issues that had cropped up along the way that were entangled with her sexuality. As these stress points were resolved, Lupa recovered, and eventually things were back to, well, as normal as things ever get for us!

One of the great things about metamorphic kink magic is that the internal skills learned can be applied outside of that context as well. A lot of metamorphic magic centers on being able to explore your own psyche, and the kink aspect helps you to be more honest about yourself sexually. These are both useful in the event that stress and other issues put the kibosh on your desire.

The solution we've worked out for ourselves, and which may work for you, is surprisingly simple in form. Get yourself into a comfortable position for meditation that you can hold for a while; or, if you prefer, go for a long walk alone in a place where you can let your mind drift without worrying about getting yourself lost or injured. Start with one simple question: Why am I stressed? Use the answer to start exploring through a conversation with yourself. Lupa will often have metaphorical conversations between her logical, rational left brain (LB) and her emotional right brain (RB). One example went something like this:

LB: Why am I stressed?
RB: Because I hate my job! Hate it, hate it, hate it!
LB: Why do you hate it?
RB: Because it's a total waste of my time. I don't want to be there.
LB: Why is it wasting your time?
RB: Because it's not what I want to be doing with my life. I'd rather be writing or creating artwork.
LB: So why aren't you doing those things instead?
RB: Because I don't make enough money freelancing yet to be able to justify not having a day job.
LB: So is there something you could do besides freelancing that involves writing?
RB: Well, maybe I could do contracted work like Taylor does. After all, he seems to enjoy what he does.
LB: Well, what's stopping you?
RB: Well, I need to work on my resume, and accentuate the writing parts, and talk to Taylor about the possibility of me getting a better job. After all, he has made the offer to me that if I wanted to get a better job he'd support me while I looked.
LB: Why don't you start on that tonight? It's better than stressing over hating your job, and you have opportunities open to you.

Not long after this internal conversation, Lupa did start on a job hunt and landed a couple of successful contracts in subsequent months. While this didn't entirely solve her problems, it did relieve a good bit of stress and helped her recovery come about that much faster.

Stress also affected Taylor, back when he was in grad school. Three months before he met Lupa, Taylor's libido took a dive and he had no sex drive whatsoever. He went to the doctor and all tests turned out fine. He was told it was probably stress. Taylor wasn't satisfied with that answer and decided to do a pathworking to find out if that was the case. Maryam (his roommate and girlfriend at the time) helped put him in a trance and narrated him through a journey where he could discover the root of his problems. As it turned out it was a combination of stress, but also some energetic and emotional blockages he had in regard to sex. One issue he had was a fear of being in a relationship where the only thing that happened was sex, as opposed to other meaningful activities. He'd been in previous relationships where he'd felt used for sex and so he'd steered himself toward relationships where there wasn't much expectation of sex.

Once he realized the root issues, Taylor could begin to work through them. He'd recently realized that he needed to make some life changes and one way of doing that involved starting a regime of Taoist meditation designed to dissolve internal energetic blockages, as well as freeing up the emotions associated with the blockages. The breathing had the added benefit of strengthening the circulation of blood for the internal organs, and the genital region.

Around the time Taylor met Lupa he'd already started noticing some effects, mostly subtle, which included some changes in his behavior and a bit less stress. Lupa added an additional element with both her patience and the BDSM play they engaged in. This allowed him to further act out some stresses and deal with them, while realizing he could also have a healthy sex life. Within a couple of months Taylor's sexual blockages were dissolved and he'd resolved a lot of the stress in his life. The regime of meditation and BDSM helped him become comfortable with his body and other aspects of his life. BDSM, when used properly, can be rehabilitative for dealing with sexual issues.

You can use breathing meditations to also help you work through BDSM burnout. You might be burned out because of psychological issues that were raised up by the kink play. The important thing to do is not avoid the issues, but work through them at your pace. Meditation or work with a therapist can be useful for processing issues that are raised up in the course of play, so that eventually you can play again without any guilt.

Final Thoughts

Metamorphic or transformative magic has many applications in kink. The use of pathworking, energy play, and invocation are all magical tools that can help a person transform into whatever s/he wishes to be. You should exercise caution, as this kind of working is powerful and intimate. You are not changing yourself alone. You could be changing someone else as well, and allowing that person an opportunity to change you. Make sure you trust those you work with in this kind of environment.

Our work of this type has been limited to each other. When others are involved, we just play. While we're intimate and open with each other, we're not as inclined to be as intimate and open with other people. If you are uncomfortable being completely honest and open with a partner, limit your kink sessions with hir to fun rather than serious work. A deep metamorphic working may be too much if you are uncomfortable. This working involves the deepest level of trust you can give.

Chapter Eleven: When Two Won't Do – Solitary and Polyamorous/Polyfuckerous Kink Magic

It takes two to tango, and two for tea is nice, but two isn't always the magic number for sex and relationships. We all go through periods, involuntarily or by choice, during which we're single. Some of you may have utterly vanilla monogamous relationships with partners that you love completely, but still want to practice kink magic. For many other people, monogamy just isn't a good fit. This chapter addresses variations on the usual two-person theme.

Lonely? Or Just Independent?

Solitary sex magic sounds impossible to many, and solitary kink likely even more so. However, as numerous chaos magicians have discovered, orgasm through masturbation is an effective way of achieving gnosis for charging sigils and other works of magic, and it's not uncommon for magicians to evoke spiritual entities for nonphysical sex.

The kink isn't too hard to add in at this point, especially for bottoms. Bondage is a good example. While it may be more fun to have someone put your collar and cuffs on you, you are capable of doing so yourself (though some styles of cuffs may be a little tricky). Gene, interviewed in *Different Loving*, described solitary business trips when he would set the lights on an automatic timer, and then bind himself with a combination lock. The lights would go out a couple of minutes later, and for several hours, until the light came on again he'd have no way to see well enough to unlock himself (Brame, Brame and Jacobs 1993).

You don't have to be that complex about it; just wearing the collar and cuffs can put you into sub space. First, test one wrist cuff at a time to make sure they're functional, especially if you're using handcuffs or other lockable cuffs, and keep the key within easy reach. If you choose to tie yourself to anything, be sure you can easily free yourself. For example, you might tie one end of a rope to one of your cuffs, thread it through an eyehook in the wall or around a bedpost or chair arm, and then keep it taut by holding the other end in your hand.

Under no circumstances should you bind yourself in a way that makes it difficult or impossible to free yourself, or in any way that restricts your breathing! The latter is a particularly important point: people have accidentally killed themselves through autoerotic asphyxiation. If you can't free yourself, and no one can hear you, the very least you may experience before someone finds you is loss of bladder and/or bowel function once you can't hold it any more. However, if you're stuck there long enough you'll end up dying of dehydration or, depending on the temperature, hypothermia or overheating. Remember that whole "hazardous to your health" thing in the disclaimer at the beginning of the book? This is definitely under that heading. If you must bind yourself without a way out, make sure there's someone trustworthy nearby who can help you in an emergency. Gene, in our example, performed his self-bondage in a hotel room where a maid would be by at least once a day, and where there was hallway traffic. A good website with ideas on creative and (relatively) safe methods of self-bondage is http://www.icebondage.net/; we recommend you take a look.

You can inflict pain on yourself in a number of creative ways. While self-flagellation sounds like fun, it can be tougher than it looks. This is one of those things where practice makes perfect. First, work on your aim so you're not accidentally whacking yourself in the kidneys full force—or causing the tips of the flogger to come around and catch you in the face unexpectedly! It's a good idea to warm up with upper body stretches; you're going to be putting your arms in strange positions repetitively, and pulled muscles are no fun.

If you can't reach your back, try striking the insides of your thighs (be careful of your more sensitive bits!) or your butt. Pinwheels and candle wax are other fun toys for self-inflicted pain. If you like non-painful sensations, ice, velvet, feather dusters, and plenty of other tangibles are available for you to use on your own skin.

You can combine any of these practices with masturbation to create sex magic. The method doesn't really matter—hands, toys, pillows, blowup dolls, whatever you use to get yourself off will suffice. We've even seen actual sex machines (exactly what they sound like).[23] Use common sense with any sort of penetrative toy—some are made of rigid plastic that isn't as yielding as flesh, so the

---

[23] Yes, we're serious. Check out http://www.bdsmstore.com/productcart/pc/cat105.asp for examples.

risk of injury is greater. Additionally, since a toy won't go soft, you can theoretically thrust until your arms get too tired. Keep in mind that your various orifices may not hold up as long!

Solitary metamorphic kink magic isn't so easy when you're the top, though you can use the ASC of top space to explore your dominant fantasies, feelings and motivations. This can touch on your deeply-ingrained imprints and conditioning. In any case, it may be a good idea to do a few solitary practice runs if you're not an experienced dominant in general, because it can help uncover unhealthy aspects of your dominant side. Turn a fantasy into a guided meditation, and explore why you're turned on by a particular act, why you may enjoy inflicting pain or having power over someone else in play. Just as the bottom is led into the deeper parts of hirself, the top touches on hidden realms of hir own psyche.

Tops may utilize invocation and evocation. Invoke before mentally working through a particular scene, and observe how the entity enhances your ideas. Another idea: evoke an entity into your mental ritual and have hir be the bottom, though keep in mind what we said earlier about entities and consent. If desired, you may evoke the entity into a pillow or other inanimate object if you wish to utilize physical flogging, though we'd imagine being evoked into a pillow probably isn't as much fun as being evoked into a warm, sexy human being. (Of course, if the purpose of the evocation is to find a human partner, the pillow evocation might strengthen your case!)

Top or bottom, your most important solitary kink magic tool is your imagination. It's crucial for anything involving visualization, whether a simple fantasy to shoot off a sigil, or an elaborate evocation of a spiritual sex partner. Make sure you put as much detail into the visualization as possible, as this will help manifest the desire into reality.

Before working solitary kink magic, it's best to gain experience with ASCs. Ground excess energy after a solitary kink magic ritual or session. Eat protein-heavy food, take a nap, or walk around your home a bit if you find yourself having a little trouble getting back into an ESC. If you aren't sure you'll be able to return to "normal," you'll probably want to practice meditating with calmer forms of trance before working solitary kink magic. ASCs can be as intoxicating as alcohol or drugs when they're intense enough, and you want to be solidly grounded before getting behind the wheel of a car, going to work, or otherwise interacting with people (other than those who are already aware of your ASC).

While solitary kink magic can be used for just about any magical purpose, many solitary kink magicians would be more interested in finding suitable partners. Before you go leaping off into love spell territory, though, here are some things to consider: If you're practicing solitary kink magic because your partner(s) happen to be vanilla or not magical (or both), you need to consider your current relationship status. For instance, if you're in a committed monogamous relationship with a vanilla or non-magical partner, then it would probably be unwise to find a kink magic partner on the sly.[24] Dishonesty damages and destroys relationships, and it wouldn't be fair to potential kink magic partners, either, especially if you didn't explain the situation to hir/them in advance. If you're seriously considering sneaking around on your significant other(s), then you should examine the health of that relationship - not another kink magician.

If your vanilla significant other(s) has no problem with the idea of you experimenting with kink magic with someone else, it's still important to communicate honestly with everyone involved (including yourself). If anyone directly involved has any problems, the issues need to be addressed thoroughly and as soon as possible. Otherwise, they may stagnate and cause worse trouble down the line.

When you are ready to find a partner for kink magic experimentation, first you'll want to make a list of qualities in your ideal partner (allowing for the fact that people are human, and keeping your list open to change if necessary). Include the usual -- personality traits, physical appearance -- along with more specific material such as duration and type of relationship, whether the person is a top, bottom, switch, etc., and even what sorts of kink magic you'd like to work with hir.

Sigilize your desire, then think of a magical experiment you'd like to try with your future partner, and masturbate to charge the sigil. Alternatively, you could evoke a deity or entity that you associate with love and/or sex, and demonstrate what you seek by performing an astral scene/ritual with hir.

It's important to keep an open mind. The biggest pitfall in love and sex spells is trying to use them to get a particular person

---

[24]As we mentioned in the sex and sex magic chapter, some people in the BDSM/fetish scene don't consider play with someone other than their committed partners to be cheating. If this describes you and your partner(s), you'll find the next paragraph to be more appropriate.

into your bed. While you can throw your efforts in that direction, one of the beauties of magic is that if you give it enough free rein in manifesting your desire, it will find the best possible outcome. This may not necessarily be what you had in mind, and you may be disappointed at first, but in the long run the magic always seems to find the best situation depending on the parameters it's given. Additionally, giving the magic more breathing room increases the probability that it will be successful. Therefore, "Get so-and-so into my bed by Saturday night" will have a worse chance of success than "It is my desire that the best partner for me at this stage of my life will draw closer to me in a positive, healthy, long term manner through this working." Additionally, bringing a specific person into your love/sex life through magic is coercive (and, according to most magicians, unethical), and probably won't result in any real connection beyond compulsion.

Be patient. We both know quite well just how incredibly frustrating being single is, especially as the weeks turn into months, and the months, well! Magic works best, in our experience, when it's allowed to flow. Taylor likens it to water — you can either try to direct it by grabbing it in your hand, or you can use the shape of your palm and the position of your fingers to change its pattern. Additionally, you can end up with what Aleister Crowley called the "lust of result" — the conscious mind so obsessed with the idea of a particular outcome that it sabotages the unconscious mind's ability to get any result, let alone the best one.

While magic is a wonderful tool to have in your arsenal, nothing's going to happen if all you do is sit around at home on your computer, reading kinky erotica and charging sigils through the wank-and-fire method. Go out and meet people whenever possible, and keep up solitary study and practice. Remember that the time you're single is excellent for working on yourself; take the opportunity to deal with persistent issues, learn a new skill, or otherwise improve yourself. Treat yourself to some small luxury (or a big one if you can afford it), and remember that it's okay to spoil yourself sometimes.

Beyond the Dyad

Polyamory is popular enough among our friends and acquaintances that we've been to parties where monogamous people jokingly wore name tags proclaiming their one-mate-only minority state. Many of the poly folk we know are also pagan and/or kinky, and kink magic is far from being restricted to only two at a time. Unfortunately, much of the available material on sex magic is designed for couples, and so poly triads and larger relationships have to get a little creative.

While we're primarily attached to each other, we do consider ourselves polyfuckerous. This means that when the opportunity arises, one or both of us may have a brief, casual fling with a friend or acquaintance. Taylor also identifies as polyamorous and so is open to more serious relationships, but up to this time (2007) we've mostly focused on building a strong foundation out of the relationship we have with each other.

As of this writing, neither of us has worked any kink magic with a third (or fourth, or fifth...) person involved. However, Dan and Dawn, who present on BDSM spirituality in the Columbus, Ohio region, have had some experience in this respect. Below, they offer an example of a poly kink experience they had:

Dan and Dawn Speak:

We mentored a woman who was dealing with traumatizing memories of her past. She had repressed them for a long time, and they were starting to come back to her in her dreams. She had symptoms of Post Traumatic Stress Disorder. She was tired of the memories emerging at random, and wanted more control over this process. We had worked with her for a few years, using Sacred Sexuality as one method to aid in her healing. Feeling comfortable with this work, she came to us and asked if we would help her use BDSM to dig deeper. We agreed, and planned a ritual involving BDSM, ritual and Reiki.

We prepared her for the ritual by hugging her and undressing her, and then we strapped her to a frame. Next, we took deep breaths, focused on her healing, and invoked the directions (quarters) and the God and Goddess to watch over the ritual. We worked on connecting to her energetically, pulling in Reiki to help strengthen the connection and help us achieve the highest good with this process. We then proceeded to flog her. We took turns flogging her, telling her it was okay to drop her walls. We asked her to trust the Goddess to give her the memories she was ready for. We told her it was okay to have walled them up for survival of the trauma, but that she was now in a safe place with a support network and it was okay to remember so that she could lay the memories to rest. Between flogging sessions, we stroked her skin, giving her more Reiki and whispering to her that it was okay to remember.

Her walls finally dropped and she became a crying mess. We took her down from the frame so that her body could relax and she could lose herself in the crying. We draped her over a footstool, made sure she was comfortable, and paddled her. She cried and cried, releasing mental toxins from her system. After a short time reassuring her that we were okay with her crying, and that we cared enough to make her comfortable, we proceeded with the ritual. In her case, crying was good. We finished by helping her rise from the spanking position, wrapping her in a blanket, and releasing the directions.

Then, the three of us cuddled on the couch while she cried on our shoulders. We gave her major aftercare, including Reiki sessions. The aftercare lasted a couple of days while she processed the memories with her therapist. (Dan & Dawn, Sacred Sexuality & BDSM Presenters – Personal Communication 1-9-2007)

In this case, two people shared the duties of topping one bottom. This seems to be the easiest group dynamic, though it's a good idea to have equal number of tops and bottoms. If there are more bottoms than a top can handle, some of the bottoms may not mentally engage in the ritual, hile too many tops can overwhelm a smaller number of bottoms or lead to bored tops. There are examples of group kink rituals in Kaldera's *Dark Moon Rising*; while these are more spirituality based, they're good references for those looking for ideas on basic ritual dynamics.

Invocation can be fun. Two or more people can invoke deities paired together in mythology; one intriguing possibility could be Ares and Aphrodite for a nice pain-and-pleasure double topping. You could take a page out of the *Essemian Manifesto* and have at least one participant invoke a deity while the rest provide worship and service to hir/them. (There's no need to limit to female deities, nor do you have to invoke deities into "matching" containers – a Goddess may be invoked by a person of any sex, for example.)

Sensory overload is easier when more than one person provides the stimuli. Flogging someone can wear your arm out after a while, even if it's just a light massage. With multiple tops, people can take turns whipping, petting, pricking, fucking, and otherwise stimulating one or more bottoms. One can imagine the massive amount of energy that could be raised by such a rite!

It's also easy to create multi-layered rituals. In *Pop Culture Magick*, Taylor described linking sigils together through the format of comic book panels. Just as separate panels in a comic book are linked together to create a story, so can sigils be connected in order to bring the story they tell into reality. A series of desired events or outcomes are sigilized, and then placed in order in comic book panels. As one sigil manifests, it aids the rest in magical success as well, in a creative domino effect.

You can use kink magic similarly. For example, let's say you have an even number of people, half of whom are bottoms. You might bind them together energetically, and physically with rope (allowing enough excess length for them to move about as needed). Paint one sigil on each bottom, preferably in a location that you won't flog but that will be visible to you, such as the lower back over the kidneys. (Or, if you don't mind cleaning your whips later, you can paint the sigil higher and flog it off the bottom.) Then charge each sigil by whipping or otherwise stimulating the bottom wearing it. You might charge all the sigils at once, or charge them successively.

The biggest challenge will be coordination. Just as poly relationships involve a greater total of communication because they involve more people, so do poly kink magic rituals need more planning. Who will be topping, and who will be bottoming? Will the ritual be practical or metamorphic? What are everyone's personal limits and experience levels? Will there be any invocations done? Make sure the entire group plans the ritual so that everyone has input. You don't have to give away all the secrets once the roles are determined, but all participants should know the basic intent and planned methods.

Chapter Twelve: Experience is the Best Teacher ~ More Examples and Anecdotes

By now you've gained a good idea of what kink magic is and how we've utilized it. You may be thinking of modifications of your own, and we encourage you to add your own creativity and kinks to the ideas we've put forth. We share these anecdotes so that you can see detailed applications of the material and use them to compose rituals of your own.

The Human Altar Ritual

In kink magic, bondage has many uses. One of our favorites is to make an altar out of the bottom. The altar can be in honor of an entity you choose for the work, including one invoked by the top. The altar may also be dedicated to the top or, as we've done, to the bottom. It can be a purely devotional altar, or it may represent a specific goal and serve as the focus of the bottom's intent. The real purpose of the altar, however, is to test the bottom's understanding of hirself. By making the bottom into altar, s/he is sanctified *and* objectified. S/he becomes an object of reverence, but nonetheless is just an object to be used as needed. Hir status as an object of worship results simultaneously in revering hir, and humiliating hir. This is useful for creating mindfuck and for throwing the bottom into a deep subspace where the top can focus hir for the magical work.

You will want to restrict the bottom's movement; you don't want an altar base (the bottom's body) that wiggles or sways. An altar that moves too much will destroy the arrangement of tools and devotional objects. Of course, this allows for punishment, which can be useful for getting the bottom to focus on hir role as altar.

Four point restraints (cuffs at the ankles and wrists) are especially useful for illustrating that loss of control[25]. Movement is already restricted, and the bottom is spread out, making for a hopefully even surface. One alternative is to lay the bottom on hir

---

[25] Depending on training, some bottoms may be well-behaved enough to stay still without physical restraints. Dire threats of punishment may be used to keep hir in line ("If you spill any of that wine, you have to clean it up – and launder the altar cloth, and give me a bath to make sure none of it got on me", etc.).

stomach and cuff hir hands together over hir head. A variation on this allows the bottom to hold tools for the top with hir legs. Have the bottom put her calves in the air. Bind the feet together and then put some of your altar tools between the feet or ankles. The top may hang the crop and flogger by their loops draped around the bottom's toes or feet. When the top wants to use one of these, s/he just pulls it off, but otherwise expects the bottom to keep the tools in the air and available.

Once you have the base of your altar set up, it's time to decorate. You should be mindful of your bottom's limits and recognize that some items may not be a good to set upon them. For instance, we would never put a candle directly on the bottom. The heat and the hot wax, as well as the potential for burns and/or a fire would be serious concerns. If you must use candles, place them on a less flammable, not living, surface. While it might be fun during scenes to place a candle holder on a bottom's body for the fear it induces, during this ritual the top shouldn't be distracted by the possibility of the candle tipping over.

You might lay a ritual cloth on the bottom. Keep hir face clear, so s/he can breathe easily. If the cloth is heavy, it may dull the sensations of the objects placed upon the altar, so choose a thin fabric.

Small ritual effects, such as a sheathed knife, small stone statues or pictures of the honored entity/person are good tools to place on the altar, as long as they aren't too heavy. For instance, you don't want to put a fifty pound statue on a bottom's stomach—it could harm hir internal organs, and it would make it difficult for hir to breathe.

Depending on the honored entity, the exact ritual tools and objects of worship will vary. If the top invokes a god, demon, angel, or other type of entity, then s/he will decorate the altar in the colors and items associated with that entity. You should research the god or entity prior to ritual, to learn the attributes and correspondences associated with it. If the entity has a favorite scent, burn appropriate incense (though not on the bottom, for the same reason as the candles). Dress the bottom in colors corresponding to the entity, as well as scented oils (though be aware that some people may have allergic reactions to certain oils; test them a day or two beforehand). Alternately, you can also paint your altar with symbols of the entity.

Use innovative ideas; for example, instruct your bottom to chant or sing to the entity. Now *that* takes dedication and makes for quite a multitalented altar! Use traditional chants, or create your

186

own. The chanting will be an excellent way of focusing the bottom's attention and energy toward the selected entity.

You can use the above techniques regardless of the focus of the altar, even if there's no external entity involved. If the top is being celebrated, then s/he is the one who gets to decide what clothing, scents and other accoutrement the bottom wears, and is the recipient of any energy and adoration the altar/bottom provides. On the other hand, a bottom's self-esteem may be raised if s/he is created into an altar of hirself, choosing what elements go into the construction. The chants are particularly good for this, as s/he is asked to chant praises about hirself! This involves hir having to express things s/he likes about hirself or about deeds or activities s/he has done; it's especially effective for pathworking rituals in which the top leads the bottom to greater self-confidence.

Human altars may also be used for purely practical magic. If you want to send someone healing energy, lay a picture of that person on the altar, and direct energy toward the image. You may also cast sigils in a similar fashion. In fact, your altar is a wellspring of energy that you may draw upon for limitless functions of practical magic!

While you may simply use the human altar as any other altar, you may also incorporate pain and sensation play. Many of the ritual instruments you use, you will not only lay on the altar, but also apply to it. You may include sex in the adorations, regardless of the recipient of the resulting energy. This will no doubt require the removal of certain altar artifacts and bondage gear, but can make a marvelous climax to such a ritual.

Oral sex seems to be a particularly worshipful activity. If the altar is created in honor of the top, the bottom can go down on the top as a form of devotion, and the quickening energy can be directed toward the overall purpose of the rite. The top can also direct hir energy to the goal through chants, looking at a mirror (and thus worshipping the self), and/or directing the energy work into the task.

A bottom may feel sacred as the recipient of such worship; again, this may require unbinding some limbs for easy access to the genitalia. The top can also force the bottom to look in a mirror and describe for the top how beautiful the altar is, while directing energy into the mirror.

Even though sex will require some disassembly of the lovely altar you've painstakingly crafted, what matters most is intent and utilizing the concept of the altar as a medium for the magic. Sex is a wonderful focusing tool as long as you keep the goal in mind building up to, and during, orgasms. If fluid is ejaculated, you can use it as a consecration or libation to the goal, either by the appropriate participants swallowing the fluid, or by making the fluid into a symbol, or by putting the fluid onto an already made symbol or artifact representing your intent[26].

Ideally, you'll strive to sustain the sex as long as possible, continuing to circulate the energy between the top and the bottom. Try to postpone orgasm, and build up the energy. When one or both participants orgasm, focus the energy raised and released through the climax on the magical purpose of the rite, whether practical or metamorphic.

Near Death Experience Human Altar Working

This is an example of a human altar working we performed. It involved providing Lupa with a near death experience by making her into an altar dedicated to her mortality.

Taylor Speaks:

I was the top for this ritual. I made Lupa into a human altar dedicated to her own mortality, because she'd been experiencing fear of death due to the recent loss of a family member. She'd never lost someone close to her in a sudden manner, and she was realizing her own mortality. I felt that this type of working would be an effective way for her to face these feelings.

I first prepped the bedroom. I unpacked the ankle and wrist cuffs, her collar, a leash, and a blindfold. I plugged in and readied the mind machine along with a CD of music that I felt was appropriate. Once I had everything set up, I walked out of the room to fetch her.

She was working on the computer. I harshly demanded she stop what she was doing. She put away the keyboard and started turning to look at me. I grabbed her hair and told her not to look. Then I gently pushed her head down to expose her neck. I placed her collar on her, telling her that I was binding her to my will. I attached the leash and explained that while she wore it, her

[26] We want to emphasize, again, that safe sex is very important. Be responsible. We, for instance, only use sexual fluids in our play with each other. With anyone else, we use condoms and other safety measures.

independence was no longer hers. Then I put the blindfold on her eyes, telling her that her senses were mine to direct. I pulled her out of the chair and marched her into the bedroom, where I threw her onto the bed.

She was lying on her belly. I got on top of her and she struggled, trying to push me off. I pulled out my knife and symbolically "cut" her throat, tracing the knife on her skin, telling her I was killing her. I assured her that her life energy was draining away through the energetic opening the knife had made. She became limp, stating she felt weak. I told her she was going to face her mortality, and that I was going to make her into an altar to her own death.

I bound her ankles with the ankle cuffs, and told her I'd removed her ability to run away. She would have to face this experience of death. I put her hands behind her back and cuffed each of her wrists. Then I cuffed the wrist cuffs together so she couldn't move her hands. I told that now that I had bound her hands, she could focus her intent only on my instructions. She was entirely mine to use, an altar to the magic I was about to perform.

I took the riding crop, my wand for this ritual, and ran it lightly over her body. When I was ready, I hit her hard a single time. This was her final death blow, I told her. I described her spirit no longer in her body, and said that I was going to drum for it, so it would know where to go. I grabbed a wooden hairbrush and gently began to paddle her ass. I slowly increased the tempo and force, providing a gradual increase in pain. I explained that her spirit was on a journey of divination, to find and bring back answers to her fears. Eventually, I stopped drumming with the brush. Her spirit was gone.

At this point, I moved on to the evocation part of the ritual. I uncuffed the metal clip holding her wrist cuffs together. I laid her on her back and removed the blindfold. She kept her eyes closed while I put the LED glasses and headphones for the mind machine on her. I turned the machine on, turning off the lights in the room. I instructed her to find, in the patterns of light in the glasses, the most ideal possible life she could have. The patterns of light were the quantum sea and she was a seafarer, seeking the best route to manifest her ideal reality. I let her journey for a time and then I inquired if she'd found it. She said she had. I asked her to describe it to me. She described what she found and I told her to bring those possibilities into her. I wanted her to merge them into her consciousness. She did this, and then asked me to stop the mind machine and music. I stopped it.

I held her for a little while. She said she felt terrible. I told her that was because her life energy was somewhere else. I then put her to bed and told her she was going to fall asleep alone, because when people die, they go alone into death, but that on the other side she wouldn't be alone. She asked me how I could do this, and I answered that she needed to experience it. She said she felt she had no control, that she'd given all of her control to me. Indeed, she had; I explained it was to teach her to trust me more. I had control, but I would let her sleep. A few moments later, she fell asleep.

The next day she told me she'd never been thrown into sub-space so abruptly. I did so to give her the experience of a sudden, unexpected death, or in this case sub-space, which was violent in its own way. She will tell you more about that.

Lupa Speaks:

This was one of the most intense rituals I'd ever done. I really haven't had much experience with Death, so when it suddenly touched me, it really shook me up. It was the first time I'd ever confronted my mortality, and I kept us both up well past midnight, four or five nights a week for several weeks, worrying over death and crying about the loss of my family member. I was not in good shape.

It really shocked me when Taylor threw me into such a heavy scene. It wasn't what I had expected when he indicated that he wanted to play, though he'd warned me that he'd be working with me on a tough subject. I wasn't sure where things were going when he put the collar on me, but it was probably one of my quickest trips into sub space — *just like that.*

Once we were into the ritual, there were moments when I was tempted to stop it. I wasn't sure I was prepared to face my mortality, but I trusted my mate to keep me safe and not push me too far, so I surrendered to his attentions and allowed him to take me into a dread situation.

I wasn't an altar in the sense that ritual paraphernalia was placed on my body. However, you know how some tops will objectify their bottom, turning hir into a table, or a footstool? Taylor turned me into an altar. The moment my power was taken from me and my will was turned toward his working (even though it was to benefit me) I knew that I existed solely for his purpose. The fact that

190

he "killed" me only added to that. No longer was I a living being; my flesh was a mere conduit for the experience my spirit was now going through.

I've only had one other personal brush with death, when I went through the skinning ritual I described in *Fang and Fur*. In that particular instance, Taylor had energetically skinned me alive as part of a ritual to Anubis that served to remind me that the animal parts in my artwork are sacred remains, not just inert materials.

In both instances, Taylor helped to facilitate my journey into the Underworld. However, while in the Anubis ritual I had been dealing with the deaths of other living beings, in this one I was facing my own mortal demise. I had been so paralyzed by this concept that it had hindered my development. By making me explore the possibilities open to me at that junction of space and time, Taylor reminded me that I wasn't dead yet, and that there are possibilities even beyond the death of the flesh.

Leaving my body and returning to it (whether it was literal or symbolic) was a novel experience for me, and it left me physically exhausted. The feeling of reentering my body surprised me, but I crash-landed into sleep a few moments after returning. The next few days saw me rearranging my thoughts on death and mortality. I had a much more positive outlook, and thereafter, we slept better at night!

Versatility makes the human altar ritual extremely effective. We've presented a few ideas here, but anyone with a desire to experiment will surely find more. The process of objectifying a person, even into a sacred object, is still a process that puts that person into a deep subspace. To know that you can't move, that you exist only as a tribute to something else, is to know that your meaningfulness is arbitrary. Such a realization is priceless, for it tests the limits of your own existence, providing a glimpse into the most secret places of yourself where you may discover what really makes you who you are.

A Captive Audience

Catharsis often seems relegated to the bottom. However, we've tried showing throughout the book that the top is just as important in ritual, and can experience growth and advancement through ritual kink magic. This includes the exploration and exorcism of unnecessary, unhealthy parts of the psyche (demons!).

Lupa Speaks:

One ritual involved a rather unexpected twist. It started out as a bit of fun, with me topping Taylor (who was being a bit of a brat). I was doing my best to subdue him, so I grabbed him by the hair and laid him down on his stomach. He complained that his back was itchy (did I mention he was being difficult?), so I decided to calm him down by rubbing some shea butter into the skin; I wanted a nice, complacent partner to play with.

As I was doing so, I started to tell him a story. I'm not even 100% sure what exactly led me to choose this, but I delved into my own history, and told him about when I was a child in kindergarten.

I was the smartest one in class, particularly when it came to reading. I was an entire book ahead of everyone else, and my teacher would come and sit with me and help me read. I liked that sort of attention. But as I grew older and went to a new school with more kids, I found that I was no longer the best at anything. This worried me; all that attention I'd received was suddenly going to someone else!

It may have been insignificant to the people around me, but it really stuck with me over the years. All through school, I pushed myself to be the best and was always frustrated whenever it didn't work. Finally, in high school, I burned out and just did the minimum I needed to get A's and B's. I managed to put forth more effort in college and graduate *Magna cum laude*, but I still wasn't satisfied.

As I told Taylor my story, I began to break apart inside without even realizing it. At the end, I fell apart entirely. I realized that one of the driving forces behind almost everything I did was the need to be the best, without question. Since I was generally in good company and so had healthy competition, I was often frustrated because there'd always be someone better than I was at anything I tried. This led to a vicious cycle - rather than working on improving, I'd give up and degrade myself because I wasn't good enough. When I got tired of that, I'd pick myself up and try again, only to be disappointed once more.

As the shell around that part of my soul cracked open, I realized how destructive this behavior was. I let Taylor up, we ended the scene, and talked about what I had gone through. I reached the conclusion that there's no need for me to compete with anyone but myself. When I write a book, for example, I don't have to compare my work with someone else's writings on the same topic, at least not in a matter of better vs. worse. My efforts are just that — mine — regardless of what I do.

The main benefit of that ritual went to the top, with the bottom facilitating the magic but not serving as the center of attention. Taylor, the bottom, acted as a distraction and a conduit to let me, the top, express what I was feeling.

A Kink Magic Rite of Passage

The rite of passage is the metamorphic magical working that's probably most often associated with kink magic, and for good reason. Kink is a wonderful tool for bringing someone through a transitional point in hir life, sparking change on a fundamental level. The rite of passage isn't necessarily a sudden paradigm shift that changes everything in the initiate's life all at once. Rather, it serves to open hir up to a new stage in hir life and prepare hir for a series of changes that will come about as a result. Just because a person experiences a rite of passage doesn't mean that the subsequent changes will be accepted, either. A person may undergo the ordeal, only to later slide back into old behaviors out of fear, laziness or apathy. However, the intensity of a well-planned rite of passage generally leaves enough of an impression to encourage the seeker to continue on hir chosen path.

Rites of passage work because they clearly delineate the shift from one stage of life to the next. The outward trappings may remain the same immediately before and after, but the change in the mind of the person experiencing the rite is impossible to ignore. Even if the impression is only subconscious, it's still powerful enough to spark a new beginning.

The dramatic ASCs of kink magic are perfect for rites of passage — for some people, anyway. The journeys into the personal Underworld create a cthonic catharsis, shedding the old skin in the depths of the psyche and drawing forth the new. The pain mirrors that of the dismemberment of the shaman, the screams of rebirth.

When designing a rite of passage, the first thing needed is a reason. Who will be undergoing the rite, and why? What will be lost, and what will be gained? What stages of life will be involved? These stages don't have to be commonly recognized ones, such as adulthood or financial independence; every moment is a potential for a chance to start over. What's important is that the reason is meaningful to the person central to the rite.

Next, the rite needs to be designed around that reason. This is where the people planning the rite get to draw on all sorts of fun things, from psychodrama to costumery to finding just the right setting. Kaldera has some excellent examples of very elaborate rites in *Dark Moon Rising*; these deal especially with mythological archetypes and motifs. Whether you design a ten-person rite with an entire floor of a house dedicated to the sacred act, or something as simple as two people in a room with a bed, what's important is that the person receiving it will be affected enough to open up to the desired aspect of hirself and let go of that which is no longer needed.

Preparations vary. An elaborate ceremony may require the individual participants to spend days or even weeks ahead of time preparing for their roles. On the other hand, a quick and simple rite may be created and performed on the spot. We've done both, and found them each to be effective, so it really comes down to what works best for the individual situation. What you *don't* want is to get a great idea for a three-hour ritual with all kinds of bells and whistles, and then decide to do it this very afternoon, thirty minutes after everyone arrives.

The collaring ceremony we discussed in the first chapter is an example of a rite of passage. Another example is the "cauldron of creation" working. The cauldron of creation is based off the *Wraeththu* series by Storm Constantine and her concept of Aruna, or sex magic. In the series, the characters find that sex magic can be used for exploration of other realities. The chakras or energetic centers of the body are used as a way of accessing these other realities.

The main energy centers of the body process energy coming from other sources, and so they function as gateways that can be opened and utilized. The gateway is usually spiral or circular. We've used the symbols for the chakras to make a connection to a given elemental plane. You can also use other symbols, such as the Kalas, for this kind of work.

Breath work is helpful for putting a person into an ASC necessary to enter into a given cauldron. You should have knowledge about the major energy center processes, to gain familiarity of the energy you'll travel to. The Earth chakra, for example, processes the elemental earth energy, so if you were to travel into that particular chakra, you could expect to work with that energy.

Sex magic is helpful for this process. The top acts as an anchor for the bottom. The bottom visualizes traveling into a chakra or other major energetic point, visualizing an open doorway to travel to. S/he uses the momentum built up by the scene and any corresponding sex to travel through the gateway to the energetic plane or cauldron of creation s/he is seeking, guided by the top.

Upon arrival, she can use the energy found there to perform the planned magical operation. Returning to our previous example, elemental earth energy could be useful for environmental action, such as helping your garden grow better. The meanings you associate with a particular gateway are the focus of any magic you do in the cauldron. The cauldron brews together the intent and desire, with the relevant energetic vibration, and projects that energy back through the gateway and into this reality so it can manifest here. This occurs when the person is brought back to hir body, so that s/he functions as a catalyst to manifest the reality.

The operation in the cauldron can be as detailed as needed. We usually find a spirit guide that represents the element and guides us while we're in the cauldron. You can do pathworkings for that particular type of energy, perform practical workings, or even heal yourself. If one of your chakras feels blocked, go into it and find out why. You can stir the cauldron, unblocking the energy so that it flows into your body again. If there is anything in the cauldron - a symbol, a memory, or something relevant to the blockage - interact with it and find out why the blockage exists. Sometimes a blockage exists because of unresolved emotional issues or fears a person has. If your throat chakra is blocked, you might have issues with communication or self-assertion. Stir the cauldron up and resolve the issue, which will then free the energy so it can go to your chakra. You can use these same techniques to heal others as well.

We've used this working as a rite of passage involving full acceptance of an elemental influence, using that influence to change stagnant aspects of Lupa's life. Below, we present our separate accounts of what happened.

Taylor Speaks:

I didn't use pain play in this topping. I wanted something more psychological and sensual. I told Lupa I was going to help her work through stagnation by introducing her to water as an active principle. I had her get a cup of cold water and put the cup on the dresser. I then lay her down on the bed and put her arms in bondage cuffs. I cuffed her wrists together with a wrist bar and attached a clasp to restrict any movement.

I wanted her to focus on the sensations of water, but I didn't blindfold her. Having her hands bound was enough because it limited how she would feel the water. I traced the second chakra symbol in water, just below her navel. She complained of the cold, but I told her to focus less on the cold and more on the sensation of feeling water on her body.

I took a small gulp of water, and holding it in my mouth, kissed her so she could drink the water from my mouth. This was a different sensation for her and a different way of topping her, forcing her to focus on the sensations. I dipped my finger in the water and ran my finger along her lips, leaving a trace of water on them. What she felt was water as an active principle.

I instructed her to visualize the symbol of the second chakra and enter into it to find a spirit guide. I intended to stir her water to aid her, which involved me going down on her to raise sexual energy. We used the sexual energy to facilitate a meditative state so she could go into the chakra and meet the spirit guide. After I finished oral, I initiated sex with her, still working with the principle of water. She later told me she was able to meet and gain information from a spirit guide.

Lupa Speaks:

When we moved from Pittsburgh to Seattle, I found myself unable to get back on my feet, even after we were both employed and living in our own home. While I was able to write at times, my focus was *A Field Guide to Otherkin*, which primarily involved research rather than additional writing. My magical practice was almost nil, and my artwork was suffering, as well. Even our sex life suffered, though not as severely as our other pastimes. In short, I felt apathetic and unmotivated.

This surprised me, because I had come to the Pacific Northwest expecting amazing things. Here was this city that had called to me for nearly a decade, full of magical, kinky, subcultural people, a relatively progressive political atmosphere, and all sorts of quirky, independently owned shops and restaurants to explore. There were mountains all around, and large bodies of water, and a wolf sanctuary less than 100 miles away. I could share it all with my mate. What was not to love?

There was the rude awakening that all was not perfect. The cost of living is high, and the traffic's a bitch, even on a good day. It takes forever to get from point A to point B, and even longer if you want to get out of the city. These are normal things in large cities, and shouldn't have continued to keep me down once we found reasonable solutions. But my mood did not improve.

It took months for me to realize that I was in the infamous Long, Dark Night of the Soul, a stage in which many magicians find that formerly productive aspects of their lives come to a screeching halt. I found myself plunged into stagnation, and rather than taking advantage of the quiet to examine myself, I'd been running in circles trying to find a way out.

The cauldron of creation ritual was a major impetus in getting me going again. I'd recently completed a year-long dedication to the element of Water, and so we focused on the concept of flow. As Taylor reintroduced me to Water, I was able to meet with an elemental and get a crucial piece of information for my development. Soon after, I began recovering from my stagnation, and while the process took a few months, this particular ritual was the catalyst that got me going again.

Ritual Humiliation

We've worked with ritual humiliation. "Ritual humiliation is a stripping-down of the soul; it asks the question, What are you when all of this is taken away? Who are you now? The idea here is to find some part of yourself that does not leave when all of these labels are temporarily rendered meaningless" (Kaldera 2006, p. 143). Ritual humiliation can be useful for helping a person dissolve stagnation or break through the boundaries of the ego. It can take a variety of forms. In one of our sessions, Lupa needed to break down past conditioning that was interfering with her self-perception and with other aspects of her life as a result.

Taylor Speaks:

In this ritual, I used the sticky energy technique. This involved applying a bit of saliva mixed with energy on each of her hands, and then sticking her hands to a surface (Kaldera 2006). I put Lupa's hands to the wall on either side of the mirror.

I began lightly slapping her ass cheeks with the paddle. I increased both the tempo and force, while channeling an entity that

I call the Flail of the Gods. This entity, drawn from my own personal mythology, spoke loudly in a more masculine voice than my own. His eyes appeared darker. When I looked in the mirror, they appeared brown at times. While the physical color does not change, solid magic can cause one's perception to shift dramatically. The Flail of the Gods questioned Lupa about her guilt over failing to fulfill the expectations of others. Every time she tried to avoid the issue, I would step up the whipping until the pain wore her down, though she never called her safe word. Once she admitted her feelings of guilt, we explored her reasoning, with me pointing out the weaknesses in her arguments. I had her speak to her image in the mirror, and verbally forgive herself. She opened up to the one person who could help her through this: her. When she was ready to let go of the guilt, I touched her head and shoulders with the riding crop, as if I was knighting her.

We repeated this routine with three related issues. She was unable to free her hands from the wall, no matter how hard she tried. It was only when we addressed her fear of humiliation, that she broke free and tried to claw me. When we examined that issue, not only did I flog her, I pointed at her and laughed in a loud, exaggerated voice. Being laughed at made her angrier than anything else, and gave her the strength to break those energetic bindings. My topping her allowed her to face the issue instead of avoiding it. She concluded by claiming Pride for herself, something she'd never done before.

Over the next few weeks, I noticed a quiet and subtle change in her. She was more confident and less apologetic. She reacted more calmly to upsetting situations and took better control over them.

Lupa Speaks:

This particular ritual was a follow-up rite of passage to the Cauldron of Creation. While that rite loosened the stagnation and started the flow, this one blasted the floodgates wide open.

I called the quarters and evoked the Friends, Family and Guardians (FFG); then Taylor energetically/psychologically bound my hands to the wall and proceeded to flog me while invoking a being that called himself the Flail of the Gods. Whether this was an external being or just a sliver of Taylor's psyche doesn't matter; what he represented for me at that moment was the voice of all I held sacred, my FFG.

One issue I'd been working on was guilt over my lack of an active spirituality. Sure, I work magic, but at this point, I didn't have a regular spiritual practice (which probably contributed to the Long, Dark Night of the Soul). However, I've never been very consistent in my routines. I felt bad, like I was taking advantage of the FFG, who patiently help where they can. However, during this time, whenever I asked them about it, they told me to go my own pace; I'd occasionally receive a gentle reminder from one that perhaps s/he could help me with a particular situation, but no one ever demanded any sort of regular observation.

A huge load of guilt remained, compounded by my guilt over not fulfilling the expectations of others, and so guilt was the first issue brought to my attention. Taylor/the Flail used pain and sensation to wear me down until I would admit to the guilt I'd hidden due to fear judgment, and we examined it together. Then he led me to the reasons for the guilt, and to examination of what it had done to me.

I looked in the mirror on the wall before me, and I saw just how tired and worn I was. Huge dark circles under my eyes, lines on my face where they hadn't been, body sagging and unconditioned and out of proportion. This wasn't just illusion, either--I was seeing the physical damage that the psychological stress had contributed.

He ordered me to tell my reflection that I no longer needed that guilt, and to apologize for putting myself through that. It wasn't easy, because I'm conditioned to hang onto it as a defense: "See? You don't need to be mad at me, I already feel guilty!" But I did it. I let go of the guilt I felt just for *being myself,* and it felt as if a huge weight had been lifted from my whip-reddened shoulders.

But it wasn't over yet. Next, we examined the expectations of others and their effect on me, and my neglect of my own desires and needs. The trouble with expectations is that they put you into someone else's parameters, not your own. Granted, this is somewhat necessary for communication, but I'd been trying to change myself, not to what I wanted to be, but to what I thought others wanted me to be -- and in conjunction with guilt. ("Maybe if I please others, I won't feel so much guilt.")

He whipped me until I could apologize to myself for allowing others to pigeonhole me, and promise to follow my own standards-- to thine own self be true, and the only person whom you can consistently please is yourself.

The third issue was trust. I didn't trust myself to self-impose limits, so I used the limits prescribed by others. I learned how this had contributed to my ill health, and learned that I needed to trust my own decisions. I made the agreement with my reflection.

Then we got to the big one.

Humiliation.

This was the pinnacle of all the issues. Taylor/etc. began to laugh at me, telling me how worthless I was, how he didn't like me and, as a matter of fact, nobody liked me. This triggered deep issues implanted by my peers, beginning in my early childhood — I'd never been popular, and I was a common scapegoat for other kids. This left me with some very deep scars. The humiliation was the worst, because it was based on rejection. Fear of humiliation led to an inability to be myself .around others. To avoid humiliation I tried living up to the expectations of others. I kept myself in line with a steady diet of guilt, feeling additional guilt any time I displeased anyone or diverted from my assigned roles.

I'm not yet ready to reveal the deepest parts of this, but I claimed Pride as my own. I had been terrified of doing so, because my experience taught me that Pride equals hubris equals the thought that "somebody's going to cut you down to size because you deserve it, you little bitch." I'd never been very proud of myself; on the rare occasions I felt pride, I overcompensated and bragged — I'd had little practice, after all. I almost didn't take Pride, that night. But then I had an epiphany.

I am a Magician. I realize my power to shape my reality to my desires. I am not a lesser or greater being than anything else in my reality, only different. Gods may have more power in some ways, but they aren't better than I am, nor am I better than they are, or better than a rock, or a shoe, or a molecule of water. Hierarchy is something artificial and illusionary; everything within my reality is equally important to its makeup. Some may have more immediate effects on me than others, but they're no better.

I am allowed to be proud of myself; there's a lot to be proud of. That doesn't mean I have to be arrogant, though some people would label being openly proud in any way as arrogance. I've spent too long with the Church, peers, and society in general telling me that it's wrong to be proud. Well, you know what? Feeling guilty all the damned time hasn't helped me in any way, so why should I continue to feed something that is obviously harmful?

Guilt is not the same as concern and respect for others. I don't mind feeling concerned about my effect on someone else. However,

I am deprogramming the guilt for simply being myself. I'm tired of walking around worrying whether I'll say or do something to offend someone, and therefore make them dislike me or say mean things about me. Feeling remorse over, say, beating the crap out of someone is not the same as being guilt-tripped for having an opinion or disagreeing with another person.

I emerged from my ordeal relieved of guilt. Not just the old Catholic reconciliation in which I tell all about the bad things I did and promise not to do them again, but going in and excising the source of unhealthy guilt. Time will tell whether we need to go back in and do more work. All I'm going to say now is--I feel a hell of a lot better.

It may seem ironic that a ritual designed to inspire humiliation led Lupa to pride. However, the things we fear most often hide our true strengths from us. Submission is often a strength rather than a weakness -- it is the ability to completely accept the situation for what it is, rather than placing expectations upon it. Within that state of dual detachment and awareness, it is possible to explore areas of ourselves we might have been unwilling to touch otherwise. The guilt and shame others place on us are what keep us supposedly equal to everyone else. In the guilt-trippers' minds, these boundaries serve to keep us from dabbling in the occult or in weird and "perverse" sex acts, and from harming ourselves by biting off more than we can chew; we remain "equal" in that we don't sink any lower than the rest of society. What we have found, however, is that this "equalization" serves to keep us from ascending as individuals and developing into who and what we want to become.

Many of us who practice magic and/or kink have had to struggle with these feelings of guilt and shame for daring to indulge ourselves in "sin" and "evil." Yet within our explorations of ourselves, given a truly honest look in the mirror, we find that what is off-limits is actually that which saves us. By accepting that kink and/or magic are what we truly desire, and through educating ourselves honestly and critically, we're able to sidestep the potential pitfalls of these practices. Yes, there is risk involved in kink and magic—but there's risk involved in crossing the street, or eating a new food that you may be allergic to, or using power tools, or leaving your car in a parking lot at night. But these mundane activities each serve a purpose, and so do kink and magic. Granted, the purposes may tend to be more esoteric and less tangible. But what good are you to anyone, especially yourself, if you're trying to force yourself into a role or definition that just doesn't fit? Accepting who you are and working within those parameters is healthier than denial. Repression is unhealthy on all levels, and guilt and shame only enforce that repression.

Knowledge truly is power, and by shedding the chains of guilt and shame, we're able to open ourselves to that education. The true risk is ignorance; a little knowledge is a dangerous thing, but additional education diminishes that risk. You probably have at least one or two stories about newbies who screwed themselves (or others) up with kink or magic because they dabbled, or attempted to do too much with too little information. Maybe it was the green "dominate" who went to a dungeon and tried to get anyone with a collar to immediately bow before hir, and then took someone home and landed hir in the hospital with a couple of fists to the kidneys in an attempted scene. Or perhaps it was the brand new magician who decided to call on Loki for a love spell, only to find that every date s/he had for the next six months either canceled or went horribly wrong.

Bad things happen, but so do good things. If you never actually try what you desire, how will you know if it's for you? Furthermore, if you never move beyond safe, known parameters, how will you grow and expand?

Kink magic is an excellent tool for some people to explore and expand both the personal microcosm and the greater macrocosm. By allowing ourselves flexibility in our worldviews, we learn more about what makes us tick than we ever imagined. It takes courage to challenge our preconceived notions and society's restrictions. This is how *we* got to where we are today.

Afterword

We've presented in this book our experiences and suggestions regarding kink in magical practice. Yet in the end, the people involved are what make magic work. We are fortunate to have found each other, and to share common ground in both practices. We have developed a level of communication and honesty that is necessary for our magic to work, and for kink to be effective on all levels.

Our hope is that you can find a kink magic partner or partners, if you aren't already so blessed. Remember that communication and trust are essential. Through this path, you and your partner(s) can have intimate, vulnerable moments with each other and with whatever entities you choose in your work.

We hope you will experiment with our ideas and develop your own. While we've presented our own experiences here, they shouldn't be taken as gospel. We want to inspire you to be innovative with your kink and magic. Below we've included a few appendices with further ideas and approaches. We hope you'll find them insightful and useful in your journey.

We also invite you to visit http://www.kinkmagic.com periodically, as we post articles and other resources there. Our main website is http://www.thegreenwolf.com; you may contact Lupa at whishthound@gmail.com and Taylor at taylor@spiralnature.com.

To contact Naryu, the cover artist, visit http://www.spirit-fox.com. To contact Daven, guest essayist, visit http://davensjournal.com. To contact Dan and Dawn, guest essayists, visit http://www.bluecatservices.org. To contact Dossie Easton, foreword writer, visit http://www.dossieeaston.com.

Appendix A: The Wolfpack Dynamic in BDSM
By Lupa

Humans are animals, and therefore as much as we'd like to elevate ourselves above the "lower" beasts, we share much in common with them, not only genetically, but also behaviorally. Of all the animals that we share the Earth with, few evoke such strong reactions from us as *Canis lupus*, the grey wolf. It's theorized that when humans began developing as predators, they also started the slow process of domesticating wolves. In the generations it took for this to occur, humans observed their furry neighbors and improved their understanding of how wolves interact together. Since wolves are highly successful hunters and family animals, they were perfect teachers for humans to learn survival and social skills. While hierarchy was a part of humanity (as it is with all social primates), the adaptation of these skills from scavenging to hunting was likely aided by wolves.

The tendency to create social hierarchy expresses itself in diverse manners within humanity. We enact these roles on a daily basis throughout our entire lives. Think of how you acted towards your parents as a child versus how you interact with them now. Compare how you view friends and how you view coworkers, including your boss and anyone you may manage. Chances are that in all of these relationships there is a hierarchy, even if it is subtle. Generally, these hierarchies are accepted and integrated into life without a single thought. Frustration at being in a lower position may result in venting, though few ever try to change it in any significant manner.

There are, however, certain situations in which the hierarchy is much more pronounced. A headstrong child conflicts more frequently with hir parents or teachers, and therefore the adults put extra effort into clarifying who's in charge. A confrontation with a threatening person creates a brief, but dramatic situation in which it is quickly apparent whether the targeted person is suitable prey. The military is based entirely on hierarchy and taking orders. Inhumane treatment of prisoners is a result of the belief that the incarcerated are lower than the average human being, undeserving of even basic comforts.

In all of these situations, the exchange of power is created for a particular purpose, not for its own sake. Only in BDSM is hierarchy created simply to enact a deliberate exchange of power with no benefits beyond the act itself. While there are residual psychological effects for the participants, there are no "real world" reasons, such as maintaining order in a workplace or protecting yourself from a potential mugger on the street. A BDSM scene or lifestyle exists to create an exchange of power without effect on the outside world.

So where do wolves fit into the picture? A wolf pack is structured solely for survival purposes. Through the process of evolution, wolves learned that their best chance for species survival was to live in packs. A lone wolf can only subsist on small animals and carcasses, whereas a pack is able to bring down large game. (That whole romanticized "lone wolf" idea is a myth — a single wolf trying to take down a moose is liable to end up dead.) Packs are better for raising whelps, and many wolf packs are comprised of the alpha pair plus some of their offspring from various litters. A pack can defend a much larger territory than a single wolf, which leads to more opportunities for food.

For this pack structure to work, it is necessary to determine pack order - the position of each wolf with regard to the rest of the pack. For instance, typically only the alpha male and female breed, except in years when the species' numbers are low. To earn the right to pass on their genetic material, the alpha pair establish their dominance and may intimidate the other wolves to prevent them breeding — female wolves may actually be prevented from going into heat in this manner.

The hierarchy determines when each wolf feeds at a large kill. The dominant pair feed first, followed by the rest of the pack, in descending order of dominance. The omega wolf, eating last, also bears the responsibility of caring for the pups while the rest of the pack goes off to hunt.

Fights for higher rank do occur, often when younger wolves reach sexual maturity. This results in some of the young leaving the pack to start their own families, but some remain. A wolf ousted from hir place is not chased from the pack, but simply assumes the lower position. Wolves that join the pack from outside (assuming they are accepted into the pack's territory) must also establish their place within the pack.

For the most part, the pack hierarchy is relatively stable. Fights are rare and primarily occur around breeding season. The rest of the time, pack members communicate dominance and submission on a constant basis through scent and body language, and to a lesser extent, through vocalizations. While scents are largely a mystery to humans, we use body language more extensively than we realize, and vocalization is a primary form of communication for us. Watch a submissive wolf and submissive human—both will affect "shrinking" postures, trying to appear smaller. Their voices pitch higher and more plaintively. The submissive will do hir best to stay out of the dominant's way, who in turn displays hir size and strength, often with aggressive vocalizations.

We see that there are parallels between wolves and humans with regard to social structure. It's true that we could use any number of animals for comparison. Chickens are well-known for their pecking order, and even fish in an aquarium establish territories. However, humans have a tendency to romanticize animals, and let's face it—chickens and goldfish just aren't as appealing as wolves.

Human categorization of wolf pack structure has provided us with an excellent dynamic for BDSM. While the dynamic can be applied to any number of participants, we're going to focus on three in particular: the Alpha, the Beta, and the Omega.

The Alpha: This wolf/person is at the top of the heap. S/he knows exactly what's going on at all times, and has control of the situation. While s/he may allow other members of hir pack to take control in certain situations, and will allow them to give feedback, ultimately it's hir call.

The Beta: While submitting to the alpha/dominant, the beta still maintains hir personal power in all situations outside of the dynamic. For the beta wolf, this means no wolf besides the alphas can automatically expect submission. In human terms, this submissive is someone who gives over hir power to hir partner, but only in scening; s/he retains hir own finances, personal issues, and other important life decisions for hirself. While s/he may be in a lifestyle, s/he may also only limit hir submission to scening—it all depends on the individual.

The Omega: This is the lowest ranked of all. The Omega wolf eats last and is picked on by the rest of the pack, though never driven out entirely. To hir falls the task of staying home and babysitting when the rest of the pack is off to hunt. The human slave has given up all of hir rights, even the right to a safe word, and trusts that the dominant will take care of hir, just as the Omega trusts that the pack will not drive hir off. The slave also sometimes turns over hir personal property and other responsibilities to the dominant. S/he exists solely to serve hir Alpha and will do as s/he is told, even to the point of being subservient to whomever the Alpha says s/he must. Strangely enough, though, it is the Omega wolf in a lupine pack that most often incites play; like a trickster figure, s/he causes the Alpha wolves to act like pups and creates a diversion from the usual hierarchy. What does this say of the human Omega, then?

Not every situation has to include all three of these roles. An Alpha may have a live-in Beta of hir own, but then go play with someone to whom s/he is Beta. Conversely, the relationship may simply be between an Alpha and an Omega. It all depends on how much control is exchanged among the various participants. The primary difference between the Beta and the Omega is that the latter gives up all power, while the former gives it up situationally.

Other lupine traits may be utilized in this dynamic. One wolf will lick the muzzle of another as a display of submission while laying hir ears back, tucking hir tail, and making hirself appear smaller. If Taylor is in need of reassurance, he will approach me with his shoulders hunched (it's hard for someone who's a foot taller than I am to make himself smaller!) and avoiding direct eye contact, sometimes with a bit of a whimper. He'll then either kiss or nuzzle my face or neck. A dominant wolf subduing another wolf may grasp the loose skin on the back of the other's neck in hir jaws, or place hir paw on top of the other's head or neck. In the same way, I will grab the hair at Taylor's nape if I want his attention or if he needs reassurance that I'm in charge (and therefore able to protect him).

One thing neglected in conversations about wolves is the alpha pair's submission to other wolves in certain situations. For instance, lower ranking wolves may take control during a hunt. In addition, alpha wolves sometimes play-submit to their subordinates. (Check *Of Wolves and Men* for details)

This is reflected in our relationship. I am the Alpha, while Taylor is the Beta. We're both polyfuckerous, meaning while we're monogamous to each other emotionally we'll still play with others, either individually or as a pair. Taylor demonstrates his role as Beta with his willingness to submit only to me. When playing with others, except in extremely rare exceptions, he will only top. However, both of us are switchable, and the power dynamic can vary depending on the situation. While I am the dominant, I will sometimes Bottom to Taylor in play. In cases where Taylor has more authority, such as healing and health issues, I defer to his wishes. Still, that authority stems from Taylor's desire to serve me, and my needs and desires come first.

There's a responsibility in being Alpha. It's not all about me punishing my Beta any time he displeases me. If you watch a wolf pack closely, you'll notice that the vast majority of confrontations are bloodless, albeit noisy. They sound worse than they are. Fights rarely result in serious injury, and death occurs even more rarely. Body language, perhaps with a growl or two, resolves most conflicts. It is similar with us. The hierarchy is well established and mutually consented, and most of our disagreements are resolved with words. Only rarely will any physical discipline come about, and then it's more as a catharsis for both of us once we've settled the issue. Wolves are much more peaceful than many people would believe.

As Alpha, I protect my Beta when I feel he needs backup. I trust that he can make decisions for himself—he did a good job of it for the 28 years before we met. But sometimes I have to intervene. Usually it's a situation that could affect his safety, or when he is unsure of what to do. Of course, he does the same for me, but from a different approach. Whereas I expect him to comply (though he has negotiation rights), he must petition me. These approaches tend to be subtle, but they're a definite undercurrent in our communication.

Overall, the wolf pack dynamic is subtle, as well. The participants must understand their roles in the pack and must be sensitive to even the slightest displays of dominance or submission. Ideally, status should be communicated through small cues—vocalizations and body language. This means that all participants must be familiar with each other's personalities and communication styles.

The wolf pack is not a place to be constantly challenging the hierarchy; major conflicts are reserved for serious issues. The Alpha needs to be prepared to defend hir place from any threat from below, and the Beta or Omega should not seriously challenge the Alpha unless s/he's prepared to become Alpha hirself. The power exchange can fluctuate depending on the situation, if that is preferred, but in the end, the Alpha remains the Alpha. This dynamic probably wouldn't work too well with smart-ass masochists or those who like to top from the Bottom. While it's not necessary to have an ironclad Master/slave contract in hand, the basic hierarchy needs to be clearly defined and agreed to, ahead of time.

I should also point out that wolves are not unnecessarily cruel. They establish their dominance, but they don't abuse each other. In this dynamic, if the Alpha wants the Omega to clean the kitchen, s/he does not then go into that kitchen, empty the contents of the refrigerator on the counters and floor, and then tell the Omega to do it all over again. The point is to work together, not break others down. There is a place for that kind of mindfuck, but not in the wolf pack, at least not as I interpret it.

If you want to work within a wolf pack dynamic, I recommend studying wolf behavior first. Barry Holstun Lopez' *Of Wolves and Men* is the best book to start with; it dispels misinformed notions about wolves and explores not only lupine behavior and biology, but also the complex relationship between wolves and humans. I also recommend attempting this hierarchy only with someone with whom you're in a long term relationship, as it requires that all participants know each other exceedingly well and can communicate openly about any topic that may arise. It's not necessary that everyone live together, but the wolf pack dynamic can be easily applied to a 24/7 lifestyle. It's also easy to apply outside of the home, as the cues are extremely subtle.

You can experiment with the dynamic with your own kinks as well. Personally, piss and scat hold no interest for me except as markers to measure my health by. The less squeamish, though, may try expanding into literally marking the territory. (Just please keep health hazards, particularly in regards to feces, in mind!) While I use wolves only as symbols and inspiration, I can see the wolf pack dynamic expanded into the realm of animal play.

Ultimately, the wolf pack is designed as a support system and safe haven. Wolf packs are family groups, not a network of bullies and victims. It should bring participants closer together and give them a sense of security. While wolves in the wild hunt together and maintain their hierarchy, they also spend time playing with each other and enjoying the company of the pack. It's not about who's the toughest wolf of all; it's about working together, playing together, and being there for each other.

Appendix B: Sacred Sensuality
By Taylor Ellwood

It's always struck me as odd that sensuality is downplayed in sex magic, and in sex. In the various books I've perused on sex magic, I've seen little mention of sensuality, as if it's something unspoken and implicit in sex. While these books explain that the sex act is not just about the physical body or that use of different muscles will greatly aid the sex act, they don't focus on sensual intimacy. Too much focus is on the act of sex, specifically the physical penetration. The attention of the heterosexual culture hovers around the steamy moist hole of the pussy (or the other waiting orifices) and the hard, rigid, pulsing penis. This attention has made these organs virtual entities in and of themselves, separate from the bodies they happen to inhabit. The focus is on satiating these independent entities and reaching the big O. There are stereotypes that go along with these organs -- that a woman should always spread her legs, that a man is always hard and ready to go, and that every time you start to be intimate, it must lead to sex.

There's another assumption associated with sensuality: that only women are sensual. All women are supposed to be in touch with their bodies and able to do sexual acrobatics because of how sensuous they are. Men, on the other hand, apparently only want sex and don't appreciate the sensual nature of the body.

The problem with the stereotypes is that they are unrealistic and used to pressure people toward a detached perspective about sex, namely that you get in, do it, get out and go on with your day (or a thrust and a grunt, as I call it). Not every intimate encounter needs to end in sex; not everyone is ready to go 24-7, and *everyone* has the potential to be sensual.

To experience sacred sexuality, it's important to experience sacred sensuality first. Sacred sensuality involves getting in touch with your body -- and not just the genitals. It emphasizes the importance of *all* of the senses, and using those senses to pleasure yourself or another person. It reveres each person and explores each person, putting the intimacy back into the sacred experience. It emphasizes that the act of sex, if it occurs, is not about the genitals, or even about energy work involved, but is about the entire body, the entire person, and revering who that person is and what s/he means to you.

The night I met Lupa face-to-face for the first time was a night of sensual bliss. At first, Lupa focused on coital sex, but I steered her away from it, and focused instead on sensuality. We spent the night of touching all over our bodies, breathing on the skin, using hair to tickle, and kissing in random places. It was a night of massage, talk, occasional long kisses, and focus on devotedly bringing forth pleasure to the entire body. It was also a night of pathworking, as I raised the totemic energy of Fox within her. It was a night of connection, and that connection allowed us to see each other as human beings. The fixation wasn't on the genitals or getting that brief moment of orgasm.

The problem is that the mainstream concept of sexuality is focused so much on that one moment of orgasm that we neglect the sheer pleasure of the entire human body and the intimate spirituality that we can find through the connection that such pleasure brings. Taking your time and exploring your partner's body is part of what sensuality is about. To appreciate the sacredness of sensuality, try exploring your own body first. Exploring your body means getting to know it. Lightly trace your fingers on your skin, especially parts of the body other than the genitals. Play with your hair. Don't be afraid to try rougher sensations, such as slapping. You might find you enjoy that. Pain is simply stronger stimulation and can be part of the sensual experience without any additional forays into BDSM.

Another way to explore your own sensuality is to use different objects. Run a flogger lightly on your chest or arms. Rub a piece of fur on your skin. Experiment with different foods, which can be sensual through taste. Randomly kiss parts of your body or breathe on your skin and see how it feels. This allows you to get in touch with your body and discover what sensuality can be. Ranges of sensation are amazing to feel and are often overlooked in sex because of too much focus on the genitalia.

By getting to know your own sensuality, you can show your partner what you like to feel, and turn hir on by demonstrating sensuality when you want to be intimate. Instead of focusing on the penultimate sex act, slow down. Undress each other, and appreciate the view you've been privileged to receive. Randomly start touching your partner's body. Smell your partner. Kiss hir in random places. Try to lose yourself in the moment. Don't look at the time, or think about what you need to do later in the evening. Focus on the moment and the person with you. Experiment. Try different sensations, and ask your partner's opinion of them. Whisper words of endearment and breathe on different parts of the body. Trail your nails lightly on hir skin and see how s/he reacts. Most of all, look into each other's eyes and see each other as people. If sex does occur, you'll find that the experience heightened by the sensual foreplay.

The connection you create is the spiritual aspect of sensuality. For me, sensuality is partially energy work. I'm not merely touching the person's physical skin, but also hir energy. I'll often focus not only on physical sensations, but also on energy. I enjoy using my breath to do this. Pranic breathing involves drawing the energy from the air you breathe into your body, but you can direct that energy elsewhere. I'll breathe on the skin and send the energy to the part of my partner's body that I'm stimulating. This will affect hir both on the physical and energetic levels, and can be very pleasurable.

The spirituality of sex can never be fully appreciated if it's not complemented by an appreciation for the sensual. When we learn to experience the entire sexual body as opposed to one organ, we learn that it is not about the orgasm so much as it is about the pleasure of the build-up, the journey that occurs as opposed to the brief intangible goal fleetingly experienced. Learning to be sensual involves learning to connect with your body, with your sense of self, and then learning to share that with someone else. That is a gift of magic, in and of itself, for when you share yourself with someone, and open up to that person, you discover that the mysteries of sex magic are not found merely through raising your energetic levels until you blow your seventh chakra out. You find them in the depth of the connection you create with someone. Sensuality is the key to the door. Open the door and explore the connection you can have, through the softest of touches, the wisp of breath, and the gaze of eyes that drink in the sight of you in full appreciation of your entire body.

213

Appendix C: The Bondage Tarot Spread
By Daven

For some time I have been trying to reconcile BDSM and paganism. About two years ago, I really started focusing on this quest. The Bondage Spread is designed to show what forces or combination of things the querent is doing which are holding them back from their goals and dreams. Needless to say, this is a very direct and plain spoken spread.

This is based on the model of a "Saint Andrew's Cross", a device on which the submissive is tied in an X shaped position. Normally the back is exposed and this is used to flog or punish the submissive. A flogging will normally focus on the back, the buttocks, and the backs of the thighs, either for pain or for a meditation.

Just as a personal observation, I have been tied in this position and had very deep meditative experiences during a flogging session. It can be very cathartic experience if it is done correctly, not only from the trust given to the person doing the flogging, but also from the vulnerability. Laid out according to the diagram the meanings and positions are these:

Cards 1 and 2, The Left Hand: This represents the power others hold over the querent

Generally this includes the people on the outside of the situation who are holding the querent back in some way, be it bosses, family or friends, to give some examples.

Cards 3 and 4, The Right Hand: The power the querent has over themselves

This was to be what the querent is doing to hold themselves back, but it has changed in practice to be the abilities and talents they have that are directly relevant to this situation. These can be helpful talents, or things that hinder the querent, like bad habits.

Cards 5 and 6, The Left Foot: Decisions in the past that others made that affect the querent still. This can be a decision made that has direct bearing on the situation the querent finds themselves in. For example, an employer may have made a decision in the past to only offer certain healthcare benefits to their employees and that decision can be affecting the querent now. In general, this is any decision that has direct bearing on the question that the querent did not make, including decisions they didn't even know about.

Cards 7 and 8, The Right foot: Decisions the querent made in the past that are still affecting them. Generally speaking these are only decisions that have bearing on the matter at hand. A financial problem that is caused by lack of foresight in credit would show up here, but not necessarily a student loan taken out a long time ago and paid back.

The "Feet" seem to be related to a point. And they generally show things like college or childhood and other decisions from quite a long time ago. I've been seeing a lot of student loans and financial strife here when I do these readings. But I have also seen other things like pregnancies and so on. The key to these two segments of the reading is that it is a set of decisions that is directly affecting the querent's life **right now**. Having to pay back a student loan may not show up as anything, but a pregnancy that resulted in a child who is currently in the hospital will show up like this.

Cards 9 and 10, The Head: Restraints the querent intellectualized into being.

This and the next pair of cards are about the querent themselves. This tends to be the "excuse" section. All of us rationalize behaviors into being simply by thinking about it, and those excuses tend to be restraints that are taken on very willingly; thus they are hard to get rid of. It's one thing to subconsciously know about these, but it's another to be told that this is directly holding the querent back from something.

Cards 11 and 12, The Belly: Restraints the querent emoted into being.

Same as with The Head, but just a level or two down. Things like getting a broken heart and deciding in the throes of recovery to never love again are included here. This is specific to the emotions, however, and they tend to be buried deeper in the querent's psyche and thus harder to correct.

Left Side: Outside Influences
Right Side: Internal Influences

The same cards are reinterpreted in the context of these new groups and with the "spin" of the position to give new insight and meaning to them.

Both sides are important. The outside influences are forces at work from outside of the querent that have a direct bearing on the restraints the querent wears. It is pressure from work, family, time and money. The right side is what the querent is doing **that is causing a reaction which is holding them back** from the outside. So instead of having a card that says they are too arrogant, they may have a card that says that because they are getting in everyone's face and gloating, it's hurting other's feelings and that is causing them to be resistant to helping the querent. It's a subtle difference, but it is critical.

Cards 13 to 17, The Breakout

These five cards taken together tell the querent how to escape the bonds they find themselves in. It is not fun, it is not kind, it is very "in their face", and generally obvious advice that is found in the rest of the spread will not be repeated here. A card saying that they are too free with money and that they should hold on to it will not be stated here again. Instead they will get something that has a direct bearing on the situation through action the querent can take.

Please note, that this is very much a means to an end. It cannot be interpreted as a 1-2-3 path to success, but more as a "these are things you need to think about and work on in order to fix the situation". The cards can be looked at as a group, individually or as specific advice. The important factor is to remember that this is how to fix the situation.

As stated, problems that show up in the main reading won't be repeated here. A problem with arrogance won't show up if it is in the main reading, but advice on apologizing and waiting out the storm this apology will cause might be.

Any card on the table can be clarified with a three-card drop. Simply select the card that is ambiguous and lay three cards above it. Those three cards should be able to clarify the confusing card, giving more depth.

The Root: Bottom Card in the Deck

Occasionally when I do a spread I will check the bottom of the deck to see if there is something else to be learned. I tend to see this card as "the root of the whole problem".

If you, as the reader, look at the bottom of the deck and the card "tells you" that it has relevance to the reading, then the root of the problem, the one thing that all the rest of these restraints spring from, will be shown here. For instance, the Queen of Swords may be here showing that all of the problems the querent is having are directly related to a bitchy woman in their life.

In testing this spread for friends, I probably did more than 40 readings using this spread. In every case where I got feedback on the spread and how accurate it was, the accuracy was very high. The querent was able to easily see things holding themselves back and keeping them from achieving their stated goal. I even heard back from a few later talking about how they had implemented the advice given and how they had overcome the problems they had which prompted the reading in the first place.

Given the cathartic nature of a Saint Andrew's Cross, the spread itself tends to not hold back. If the problems are coming from the user being an idiot, it will say so rather than hedge the advice with things like "you may want to think about...." If you find your cards screaming at you about the querent now you will know why. I was personally shocked as to how blunt my cards became.

Appendix D: The Sacred Switch
By Taylor Ellwood and Lupa

As we stated earlier, anyone can perform kink magic. It doesn't matter whether you're straight, gay, bisexual, pansexual, etc., whether you're cisgendered (identifying with the sex you were born as), transgendered, male, female, intersexed, and so on—and it doesn't matter whether you're a bottom, top, dominant, submissive, or anything other label we could stick on you.

This isn't an essay about how the switch is a superior kink magician. Rather, it's a discussion on how switching has been a major advantage for us in developing our practice of kink magic. We invite you to consider our ideas, just as with the rest of the book, and use or discard them as you see fit.

One of the primary purposes of magic is conscious change. We've both benefited from using magic as a tool for deprogramming bad conditioning, for exploring hidden parts of our psyches, and for bringing about positive developments in our lives. As magicians, we value adaptability very highly—the world around us is ever changing, and we must be mutable enough to answer those changes. Or, as Lupa likes to put it, "Stagnation equals death — keep moving!"

Switching works nicely into this paradigm, because it is so adaptable. A switch can be either top or bottom—or both in one scene, if that's what's called for. There are benefits to each side of the equation, and we enjoy being able to work with them all.

The top, for example, isn't just the person guiding the bottom through mind-blowing experiences. Topping involves ASCs of its own, and accessing aspects of yourself that you might have not realized were there. Lupa never considered that she was capable of topping until she met Taylor. Because she was so strongly conditioned to bottom, and because her other partners had been either tops or vanilla, she assumed that if there was anything toppish in her, it wasn't enough to actually take on that role. Lo and behold, though, she found herself becoming an aggressive, sadistic, cruel being in play, something she hadn't even realized was in her normal, (relatively) harmless self.

Topping in kink magic allows you to explore control issues from a different perspective. It's not all about flogging someone until they achieve gnosis. There's a certain amount of responsibility and care above and beyond BDSM play; you aren't affecting someone for the limited duration of the scene—you're causing a permanent shift in hir psyche. While this sometimes occurs unintentionally, it's part of the metamorphic aspect of kink magic. Realizing that you are orchestrating an important rite of passage in someone's life is no small thing, and if you thought you were incapable of such power and responsibility, once you're adept at opening you may very well find out otherwise!

Bottoming is about giving up control. That's a terrifying thing for many people. We like having control, or at least thinking we do; it gives us a nice, safe sense of security. Bottoming reveals that security is illusory, through a ritualized format rather than a natural disaster or serious injury. Realizing that security is a concept used to inspire calm is empowering; when you have a major change in your life, such as an accident, you're able to keep a better perspective because you realize that you really haven't lost as much as you thought you have. Change is no longer a shock, and you're better prepared for it.

We suspect that at least some of the uber-doms we've met who swear that they'll never submit are afraid of submission. This is a good reason for them to try it! Many people have issues with submission and dominance. Even Lupa, as we write this, still struggles with the idea that she actually enjoys giving up control and doing things considered undignified in everyday interactions with people. She continues to access this part of herself because to suppress it would only manifest it in harmful, chaotic ways.

The value of switching is that it allows each person to experience bottoming *and* topping. Mutability and adaptability are essential parts of a switch, because at any given moment, the switch can change from top to bottom. This isn't to say that people who prefer the roles of top or bottom don't experience mutability and adaptability, but the switch is in the unique position of experiencing both roles, and this shapes how s/he plays. It can also shape how s/he does magic in a kink scene, because s/he could play either role.

You can apply these principles to other areas of your sexual life. Sexual orientation is a good example. Contrary to popular belief, while some people fix on one orientation throughout their lives, others are more fluid. Joshua Wetzel even recommends shifting your sexuality over a notch as a way of breaking out of your tunnel vision (2006). You could also try altering your spiritual gender. Work with your animus if you're female, or your anima if you're male, or otherwise access your sexual "opposite" and bring it into full balance with what you consider to be your primary identity. You can even make love to your sexual opposite as a way of helping you balance your identity. Your spirit is not as limited as your flesh.

To us, magic is a fluid experience. Kink magic offers numerous opportunities for growth, both pragmatically and spiritually. To cut ourselves off from one role or the other necessarily limits the potential benefits available.

The only limitations we have are those we place upon ourselves. Modern occultism has shown that any aspect of a person, with enough time, will, and effort, can be modified. One of the beauties of kink magic is that it can open you up to parts of yourself you never even knew were there, and give you a context in which to explore them in a controlled environment. The things we push away hold pieces of ourselves that terrify us, but which control us in silent ways nonetheless. Embracing that which is Other can allow us to pull the veils from our fear, look it in the eye, and realize that we no longer need to give it power. And that is true liberation.

Bibliography

Books

Anonymous. (1996). *Thee psychick youth manifesto*. Sine Nomine Press.

Anonymous. (year unknown). *Essemian manifesto: Female dominance and fetishism as a religious philosophy*. El Cerrito: Self-published.

Ashcroft-Nowicki, Dolores. (1999). *The tree of ecstasy: An advanced manual of sexual magic*. York Beach: Samuel Weiser, Inc.

Bardon, Franz. (1999). *Initiation into hermetics*. Salt Lake City: Merkur Publishing, Inc.

Belanger, Michelle. (2004). *The psychic vampire codex*. York Beach: Red Wheel/Weiser LLC.

Bell, Catherine. (1992). *Ritual theory: Ritual practice*. New York: Oxford University Press.

Bell, Catherine. (1997). *Ritual perspectives and dimensions*. New York: Oxford University Press.

Black, S. Jason. (2004). Introduction. In Lisiewki (author). (Pp. 11-23). *Ceremonial magic & the power of evocation*. Tempe: New Falcon Press.

Bonewits, Isaac. (1989). *Real magic*. York Beach: Samuel Weiser, Inc.

Brame, Gloria, William D. Brame, and Jon Jacobs (1993). *Different loving: The world of sexual dominance and submission*. New York: Random House.

Brennan, Barbara Ann. (1987). *Hands of light: A guide to healing through the human energy field*. New York: Bantam Books.

Carrellas, Barbara. (2007). *Urban Tantra: Sacred sex for the twenty-first century*. Berkeley: Celestial Arts.

Carroll, Peter J. (1987). *Liber null & psychonaut: An introduction to chaos magic*. York Beach: Samuel Weiser, Inc.

Carroll, Peter J. (1992). *Liber kaos*. York Beach: Samuel Weiser, Inc.

Chia, Mantak. (2005). *Healing love through the Tao: Cultivating female sexual energy*. Rochestor: Destiny Books.

Chia, Mantak, & Abrams, Douglas. (1996). *The multi-orgasmic man*. San Francisco: Harper Collins Publishers.

Chia, Mantak, & Winn, Michael. (1984). *Taoist secrets of love: Cultivating male sexual energy*. Santa Fe: Aurora Press.

Crowley, Aleister. (1994). *Book IV*. York Beach: Samuel Weiser, Inc.

Cunningham, David Michael, Ellwood, Taylor, & Wagener, Amanda. (2003). *Creating magickal entities.* Perrysburg: Egregore Publishing.

Dan and Dawn Sacred Sex and BDSM Presenters (Personal Communication, January 9, 2007).

Dawn, Crystal & Flowers, Stephen. (2001). *Carnal alchemy: A sado-magical exploration of pleasure, pain, and self-transformation.* Smithville: Runa-Raven Press.

Easton, Dossie, & Hardy, Janet W. (2004). *Radical ecstasy.* Oakland: Greenery Press.

Easton, Dossie, & Liszt, Catherine A. (1995). *The topping book.* Oakland: Greenery Press.

Eliade, Mircea. (1957). *The sacred and the profane: The nature of religion.* San Diego: Harcourt, Inc.

Ellwood, Taylor. (2004). *Pop culture magick.* Stratford: Immanion Press.

Ellwood, Taylor. (2005). *Space/Time magic.* Stratford: Immanion Press.

Ellwood, Taylor. (2007). *Inner alchemy.* Stratford: Immanion Press.

Farrell, Nick. (2004). *Magical pathworking: Techniques of active imagination.* St. Paul: Llewellyn Publications.

Feuerstein, Georg. (1998). *Tantra: The path of ecstasy.* Boston: Shambhala Publications, Inc.

Filan, Kenaz (2007). *The haitian vodou handbook: protocols for riding with the lwa.* Rochester, Vermont: Destiny Books.

Firefox, LaSara. (2005). *Sexy witch.* St. Paul: Llewellyn Publications.

Frantzis, B. K., (2001a). *Relaxing into your being: Breathing, chi & dissolving the ego.* Berkeley: North Atlantic Books.

Frantzis, B. K. (2001b). *The great stillness: Body awareness, moving meditation & sexual chi gung.* Berkeley: North Atlantic Books.

Frater U.D. (2001). *Secrets of western sex magic.* St. Paul: Llewellyn Publications.

Hine, Phil. (1995). *Condensed chaos: An introduction to chaos magic.* Tempe: New Falcon Press.

Kaldera, Raven (2005). *The ethical psychic vampire.* Self-published.

Kaldera, Raven (2006). *Dark moon rising: Pagan bdsm and the ordeal path.* Hubbardston, MA: Asphodel Press.

Karika, Jozef. (2005). How to charge sigils by porn and other nice techniques, Part I. Pp. 42-47. *Konton magazine, 2.2.*

Kelly, Aidan (1991). *Crafting the art of magic, book 1: a history of modern witchcraft, 1939-1964.* St. Paul, Minnesota: Llewellyn Publications.

Lilly, John C. (2004). *Programming the human biocomputer.* Berkeley: Ronin Publishing, Inc.

Lipton, Bruce. (2005). *The biology of belief: Unleashing the power of consciousness, matter, & miracles.* Santa Rosa: Mountain of Love/Elite books.

Lupa. (2005). Riding the red tide: Menstrual magic and the treasure of our women's Blood. Pp. 17-19. *SageWoman, 67.*

Lyesbeth, Andre Van. (1995). *Tantra: The cult of the feminine.* York Beach: Samuel Weiser, Inc.

Mace, Stephen. (1996). The subtle body. Pp. 60-68. *Addressing power: Sixteen essays on magick and the politics it implies.* Milford: Self-published.

Mace, Stephen. (2005). *Shaping formless fire: The quintessence of magick.* Tempe: New Falcon Press.

Miller, Philip, and Molly Devon (2001). *Screw the roses, send me the thorns: The romance and sexual sorcery of sadomasochism.* Fairfield, CT: Mystic Rose Books.

Nan, Huai-Chin. (1984). *Tao & longevity: Mind-body transformation.* Trans. Wen Kuan Chu. Boston: Weiser Books.

Néret, Gilles (2005). *Erotica universalis: from pompeii to picasso.* Cologne, Germany: Taschen.

O'Connor, Joseph, & Seymour, John. (2002). *Introducing nlp: Psychological skills for understanding and influencing people.* London: HarperCollins Publisher.

Randolph, Pascal Beverly. (1988). *Sexual magic.* Trans. Robert North. New York: Magic Childe Publishing, Inc.

Service of Mankind Church, the (unknown). *Essemian manifesto: Female dominance and fetishism as a religious philosophy.* Self-published.

Varrin, Claudia. (2004). *Female dominance: Rituals and practices.* New York: Citadel Press.

Wallechinsky, David and Irving Wallace (1975). *The people's almanac.* Garden City, New York: Doubleday and Company, Inc.

Wallechinsky, David and Irving Wallace (1978). *The people's almanac #2.* New York: William Morrow and Company, Inc.

Warren, John. (2000). *The loving dominant.* Emeryville, CA: Greenery Press.

Wetzel, Joshua (2006). *The paradigmal pirate.* Stafford, United Kingdom: Immanion Press.

Williams, Brandy. (1990). *Ecstatic ritual: Practical sex magic.* London: Prism Press.

Wilson, Robert Anton. (1983). *Prometheus rising*. Tempe: New Falcon Press.

Wilson, Robert Anton. (1990). *Quantum psychology: How brain software programs you & your world*. Tempe: New Falcon Press.

WitchWitch. (2006). Witch does vampire sex magick. P. 6. *Widdershins, 12.1.*

Websites

Anonymous (2006). *Blood fetish*. Retrieved January 11, 2007 from http://en.wikipedia.org/wiki/Blood_fetish.

Anonymous. Whipping therapy cures depression and suicide crises. *Pravda*. Retrieved December 20, 2006 from http://english.pravda.ru/science/health/26-03-2005/7950-whipping-0.

Fox Internet Services (2006-A). *Development of the female sexual and reproductive organs*. Retrieved January 11, 2007 from http://www.the-clitoris.com/n_html/develop.htm.

Fox Internet Services (2006-B). *Female ejaculation, the female prostate, and the g-spot*. Retrieved January 11, 2007 from http://www.the-clitoris.com/f_html/ejacula.htm.

Frew, D. Hudson (unknown). *Crafting the art of magic: a critical review*. Retrieved January 11, 2007 from http://www.gryffintower.com/kelly.htm.

Hiscock, Philip et. al (1993). *Origin(s) of "rule of thumb"*. Retrieved 6 May, 2007 from http://research.umbc.edu/~korenman/wmst/ruleofthumb.html.

Savage, Dan (2006). *Savage love: sisters and slaves*. The Stranger. Retrieved December 20, 2006. from http://www.thestranger.com/seattle/SavageLove?oid=25851.

Toke, Leslie A. St. L. (1909). Transcribed by Potter, Douglas J. *The catholic encyclopedia: flagellants*. http://www.newadvent.org/cathen/06089c.htm. Retrieved 18 December, 2006, last updated 2006.

Other Recommended Reading

Magic

Galenorn, Yasmine (2003). *Sexual ecstasy and the divine: the passion and pain of our bodies*. Berkeley: Crossing Press.

Graham, Nicholas (2007). *The four powers: Magical practice for beginners of all ages*. Stafford: Immanion Press/Megalithica Books.

Hunter, Jennifer (2004). *Rites of pleasure: Sexuality in wicca and neopaganism*. New York: Citadel Books.

Gray, William G. (1980). *Magical ritual methods*. York Beach: Weiser, Inc.

Harvey, Graham (2000). *Contemporary paganism: listening people, speaking earth*. New York: New York University Press.

Kink

Hardy, Janey W. and Dossie Easton (2001). *The new bottoming book*. Emeryville, CA; Greenery Press.

Rinella, Jack (2006). *Philosophy in the dungeon: The magic of sex and spirit*. Rinella Editorial Services.

Sensuous Sadie (editor, 2007).*Spiritual transformation through BDSM*. Fargo, North Dakota: Gracie Passette Productions.

Wiseman, Jay (1998). *SM 101: A realistic introduction*. Emeryville, CA: Greenery Press.

Index

Did You Like What You Read?

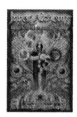
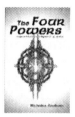
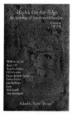
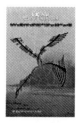

Printed in the United States
201045BV00002B/598-618/A